Tunnel Syndromes

Authors

Marko M. Pećina
Department of Orthopaedic Surgery
University of Zagreb
Yugoslavia

Jelena Krmpotić-Nemanić
Institute for Anatomy, Faculty of Medicine
University of Zagreb
Yugoslavia

Andrew D. Markiewitz
Department of Orthopedic Surgery
The Cleveland Clinic
Cleveland, Ohio

CRC Press
Boca Raton Ann Arbor Boston London

Library of Congress Cataloging-in-Publication Data

Tunnel Syndromes/editors, Marko M. Pećina, Jelena Krmpotić-Nemanić,
   Andrew D. Markiewitz.
       p. cm.
   Includes bibliographical references and indexes.
   ISBN 0-8493-6933-9
   1. Entrapment neuropathies. I. Pećina, Marko. II. Krmpotić-Nemanić, Jelena.
III. Markiewitz, Andrew D.
   [DNLM: 1. Carpal Tunnel Syndrome. 2. Nerve Compression Syndromes. WL 500 T926]
RC422.E56T86 1991
616.8′7—dc20
DNLM/DLC
for Library of Congress
                      91-26795
                      CIP

Direct all inquiries to CRC Press, Inc., 2000 Corporate Blvd., N.W., Boca Raton, Florida, 33431.

© 1991 by CRC Press, Inc.

International Standard Book Number 0-8493-6933-9

Library of Congress Card Number 91-26795
Printed in the United States
5 6 7 8 9

PREFACE

I became involved in researching the anatomical premise that leads to the onset of nerve compression in fibro-osseous and fibro-muscular tunnels at the Institute for Anatomy at the School of Medicine, University of Zagreb. My chosen field of endeavor, orthopedic surgery, took me from the institute to the Department of Orthopaedic Surgery, where I combined basic anatomical and practical clinical research about tunnel syndromes. My first publication dealing with tunnel syndromes saw the light of day more than 25 years ago.

While the inherent origin of the painful syndromes of the extremities is well known, tunnel syndromes are still neglected with the exception of some particular localizations. The intent of this book is to bring forward the possible causes leading to the onset of tunnel syndromes, impossible without the effort of the second author, Jelena Krmpotić-Nemanić, who has provided exact anatomical descriptions and drawings. The credit for the majority of the drawings and schemata goes to academic artist Edita Schubert.

My special appreciation goes to my dear friend Prof. Dr. I. Damjanov from Philadelphia, who has helped me in the selection of the third author of this book; Andrew D. Markiewitz's outstanding cooperation was highly valuable to the publication of this book in the U.S.

The publishers of CRC Press have shown a full understanding of the difficulties encountered by bicontinental authors, and they have also contributed to a great extent in the graphic design of the book. We thank them for their valuable assistance.

Marko M. Pećina
Zagreb, March, 1991

THE EDITORS

Marko M. Pećina, M.D., Ph.D., is Chairman and Professor of Orthopaedic Surgery at the School of Medicine, University of Zagreb. He is also chief of the department at Zagreb Teaching Hospital Orthopaedic Clinic.

Dr. Pećina graduated from Zagreb University Medical School in 1964. From 1965 to 1970 he was an assistant lecturer at the "Drago Perovic" Anatomic Institute of Zagreb Medical School. He obtained his M.Sc. degree in experimental biology at Zagreb University Faculty of Natural Sciences in 1968. He defended his Ph.D. in medical science in 1970 at Zagreb University Medical School. In 1970 he became an assistant lecturer at Zagreb Medical School Orthopaedic Clinic. In 1977 he became senior lecturer, in 1979 assistant professor, in 1980 associate professor, and in 1984 professor in orthopedics.

He visited and worked in many orthopedic institutions around the world for further professional training (Lyon, Bologna, Basel, London, Milwaukee, New York, Baltimore, Los Angeles, Columbus, and others). He has also participated in numerous symposia and congresses in Yugoslavia and abroad. He is actively engaged in professional association, in particular the Croatian Medical Association and the Yugoslav Orthopaedic and Traumatology Association (President 1988–1989). From 1982 to 1986 he was editor-in-chief of *Acta Orthopaedica Iugoslavia* and has since served as president of the journal council. He is also president of the *Croation Medical Bulletin* council and *Basketball Medical Journal*. He is also a member of the following international societies: International Knee Society, European Spinal Deformities Society, French Society for Orthopedic Surgery and Traumatology (Société Francaise de Chirurgie Orthopédique et Traumatologique), European Society of Knee Surgery and Arthroscopy, Italian Club of Knee Surgery (Club Italiano di Chirurgia del Ginocchio), Balkan Medical Union (Union Medicale Balkanique). He is also a member of Société Internationale de Chirurgie Orthopédique et de Traumatologie (SICOT) and is a SICOT national delegate for Yugoslavia. He is an honorary member of the Hellenic OrthopaedicTraumatology Society. He is one of the founders of the European Spinal Deformities Society and has been vice-president since 1992. Since 1990 he has been a corresponding member of the Editorial Board of International Orthopaedics.

Professor Pećina is interested in clinical anatomy and applied biomechanics of the locator system, scoliosis, knee problems, and sports traumatology. He has published more than 250 expert and scientific papers in the country and abroad.

For his professional achievements he was awarded numerous tokens of appreciation such as the Balkan Medical Union Award for Scientific Achievement. He has also received many other diplomas of foreign and domestic associations. He is a regular member of the Croation Medical Academy and an associated member of the Yugoslavian Academy of Arts and Sciences.

Jelena Krmpotić-Nemanić, M.D., D.Sc., is Chief of the Chair of Anatomy, Medical Faculty Zagreb, University of Zagreb, Republic of Croatia, Yugoslavia.

Dr. Krmpotić-Nemanić graduated in 1939 from the school for classical education in Zagreb (summa cum laude), and she obtained her M.D. degree in 1944 from the Medical Faculty in Zagreb. She received her D.Sc. in 1957 from the Medical Faculty Zagreb (1960-1963), where she specialized in otorhinolaryngology. In 1942 she began work at the Department of Anatomy as an assistant. In 1949 she became a lecturer, in 1953 and extraordinary professor, and in 1963 a full professor. From 1961 to 1980, she was the chief of the Department of Anatomy.

She is an honorary member of the Austrian Otorhinolaryngolgical Society, corresponding member of the German Otorhinolaryngological Society in Wiesbaden, Berlin, the honorary professor at the University of Munich, a member of the Collegium Otorhinolaryngologicum Amicitiae Sacrum. She is also the extraordinary member of the present Croatian Academy of Science and Arts (founded as the Yugoslav Academy of Science and Arts). Dr. Krmpotić-Nemanić is redactor of *Zeitschrift für Laryngologie, Rhinologie und Otologie*, *European Archives of Oto-Rhino-Laryngology*, and *Otorhinolaryngologia Nova*.

Among the rewards she has received are the Ludwig Haymann's price decoration, Austrian Cross of Honor (Ehrenkreuz für Wissenschaft und Kunst I. Klasse), and the Laureat of French Medical Academy.

Dr. Krmpotić-Nemanić has been a researcher and collaborator on three consecutive U.S.-Yugoslav joint board grants (N.I.H., D.H.H.S.: pricipal investigator Dr. I Kostović) concerned with the prenatal, perinatal, and postnatal development of the human frontal lobe, as well as being the principal investigator on several Yugoslav research grants.

Dr. Krmpotić-Nemanić has presented over 30 guest lectures in Europe and the U.S. She has published over 200 research papers, many of which are cited in *Science Citation Index*. She has authored and co-authored 10 books (7 of them at Urban Schwarzenberg, Springer and Delfino) and she is the reviewer of *Zentralblatt für HNO-Heilkunde*.

Her current interests include the development of the skull, paranasal sinuses, and interference of anomalies with the nervous system.

Andrew D. Markiewitz, M.D., is currently in his second year of training as an orthopedic surgeon at the Cleveland Clinic Foundation, Cleveland, Ohio.

Dr. Markiewitz graduated in 1985 from Cornell University, Ithaca, New York, with a Bachelor of Science Chemical Engineering and obtained his M.D. degree (cum laude) in 1989 from Jefferson Medical College, Philadelphia, Pennsylvania. While at Jefferson Medical College, Dr. Markiewitz received a research grant from the NIH to address cytologic staining for computer analysis, was selected honorable mention for the award Ethics in Medicine, and was inducted as a member in the AOA Medical Honor Society.

Dr. Markiewitz is currently a member of the American Medical Society and a resident member of the American Orthopedic Society. His current research interests, both clinical and basic research, are in hand and foot surgery, including fracture treatment and peripheral neuropathies.

TABLE OF CONTENTS

SIGNIFICANCE OF TUNNEL SYNDROMES

Passing through bony, fibrous, osteofibrous, and fibromuscular tunnels, nerves from their origin in the spinal cord to their effector organ risk compression, damage, and impairment of their end function. Virtually all nerves carry afferent and efferent impulses along a combination of motor, sensory, and autonomic fibers. However, patients present with signs and symptoms usually associated with the motor or sensory function of the involved nerve. Careful linking of these signs and symptoms can indicate a specific compressive or painful pathology commonly known as a tunnel or canalicular syndrome.

The expressions "canalicular", "canal", "channel", and "tunnel" have been used inter-changeably for these syndromes. Webster's proves this dilemma in semantics; *canal* and *canaliculus* infer an enclosed passage "either in bone or soft tissue," whereas *channel* is defined as a "bed where a material body may run" and *tunnel* represents a "bodily channel". In German literature, the expressions *Engpass-Syndrome, Einklemmungsneuropathis,* and *Tunnel-syndrome* compare with the English literature's *channel syndrome, entrapment compression neuropathy,* and *tunnel syndrome* or the French literature's *canal syndrome* or *loge syndrome.* All of these terms are appropriate, since they seek to describe the damage to neurovascular structures running in a common course through a small area (whether intrinsic or extrinsic in source). To simplify the discussion, this book will use the general term "tunnel syndromes", but will note the common names currently ascribed to each clinical picture.

Multiple approaches have been used to categorize the tunnel syndromes.[1] Any syndrome can therefore bear the descriptive name, which may originate from any one of the following sources:

- the compressed nerve (i.e., the ilioinguinal syndromes);
- the anatomical area affected (i.e., metatarsalgia);
- the anatomical tunnel (i.e., carpal tunnel syndrome); the motion producing the compression (i.e., hyperabduction syndrome);
- the names of the describing authors (i.e., Kiloh-Nevin's syndrome).

While the names may vary, these syndromes all originate from a lesion to neurovascular elements in a narrow anatomical space. The damage may be due to tumor compression (intraneural or extraneural), trauma (blunt, sharp, or secondary to repetitive action), infection (inflammation or actual bacterial invasion), metabolic, toxic, iatrogenic, idiopathic, vascular (ischemic,[2] aneurysmal, or tumor in nature), muscular compression, or anatomical variations.

When a patient presents with neurovascular symptoms, a careful history and physical exam must be done prior to ordering tests, scans, or studies.[3]

Pain of a radicular nature could be a sign not only of a tunnel syndrome but also a herniated disc or tumor (piriform muscle syndrome vs. herniated nucleus pulposus herniation vs. ependymoma). Raynaud's phenomenon in the hand could be due to carpal tunnel syndrome or autonomic dysfunction secondary to autonomic nerve compression. Vascular disease can lead to isolated nerve ischemia, in turn producing symptomatology characteristic of a tunnel syndrome or a combination of syndromes as in thoracic outlet syndrome, carpal tunnel syndrome, and Guyon's tunnel canal syndromes. Symptoms and signs depend on the type of nerve compressed in the tunnel: motor, sensory, or mixed. While most nerves carry afferent and efferent impulses in addition to autonomic nerve fibers, this book will follow a classic didactic approach and describe symptoms as sensory or motor. Understanding the signs and symptoms as well as the dynamic anatomy of the tunnel allows the practicing physician to identify the syndrome and promptly remove the affecting agent before irreversible damage occurs.

TABLE 1
Several Causes Leading to Alteration of Nerve Function

General categories	Compressive causes
Idiopathic/spontaneous	Fibrositis
External (to tunnel)	
Acquired	Spondylosis, arthritis, spinal stenosis, herniated nucleus pulposus
Congenital	Cervical rib
Crauma	Fracture callus, shoulder dislocations
Vascular	Aneurysms, ischemia
Inflammation /autoimmune	Viruses (measles, chicken pox, polio, diphtheria, tetanus, leprosy), tuberculosis, rheumatic disease
Metabolic	Diabetes, beriberi, pellagre, hypothyroidism, pernicious anemia, drugs (ETOH), metals/chemicals (mercury, arsenic, lead, silver)
Hormonal	Pregnancy
Iatrogenic	Casting
Tumor/neoplasm	Apial lung tumors, ganglions
Internal (to tunnel)	
Acquired	Occupation, dynamic
Congenital	Narrow suprascapular notch, anomalous musculature
Trauma	Hematoma, crush injuries, lacerations
Vascular	Aneurysm, ischemia, arteritis
Inflammation/ autoimmune	Rheumatic diseases, tuberculosis
Metabolic	lead, hypothyroidism, nutrition
Hormonal	Pregnancy
Iatrogenic	Surgical trauma
Tumor	Extrinsic (lymphomas, multiple myloma) intrinsic (schwannoma, hemangioma)

ETIOLOGY AND PATHOGENESIS

Narrowing of the osteofibrous or the fibromuscular neurovascular tunnel represents one of the major factors in the pathogenesis of tunnel syndromes. Narrowing can be caused by changes intrinsic or extrinsic to the tunnel as detailed in Table 1. These changes include tumors, cysts, inflammatory processes (rheumatic, tubercular), trauma (blunt-hematoma formation, sharp fractures), or anatomic variations. Operative exploration frequently will locate and relieve these compressive factors. However, tunnel syndromes secondary to vascular insufficiency, endocrine disease, or metabolic disturbances may not be relieved by surgical intervention. Additionally, tunnels may be compressed by anatomical variations but only when evaluated in motion. Idiopathic etiologies remain for several tunnel syndromes where extensive investigation fails to yield a cause.

Tunnel compromise does not require major changes in space to dramatically alter function.[4] Inflammatory changes resulting in slight connective tissue thickening of tendon or nerve sheaths can compress a nerve or its vascular supply. Ischemic events initially affect sensory nerve fibers.[5] If the ischemia continues, motor fibers begin to be damaged. Edema secondary to the hormonal changes associated with pregnancy, birth control pills, menopause, and hypothyroidism has been felt to cause tunnel compression. Dynamic changes of a tunnel during daily activity can create traction or compression of a nerve if slight anatomical variations exist. The variations become important because the nerve has restricted mobility between its origin and its course through the tunnel.

TABLE 2
The Difference Between Several Nerve Lesions

Nerve Lesions	Definition
Neuropraxia	Temporary loss of function (not necessarily complete) no neural disruption
Axonotmesis	Axonal and sheath disruption with connective tissue sheath preserved; recovery dependent on distance from lesion to insertion
Neurotmesis	Complete anatomical interruption of the nerve; complete loss of function; no spontaneous recover; usually secondary trauma

Nerve damage ranges from temporary and reversible to complete loss of function with or without the chance of regeneration.

Seddon[6] indicated that a tunnel syndrome could produce a neuropraxis or eventually an axonotmesis. However, complete nerve interruptions do not occur in tunnel syndrome. Recognition of symptoms may allow early intervention to relieve the compression leading to neuropraxia (see Table 2).

CLINICAL SYMPTOMS AND SIGNS

Patients present to their physician with symptoms that can range from vague complaints of diffuse pain or numbness to specific complaints of muscle weakness or of sensory changes over localized skin areas. Precise assessment of a patient's symptoms yields a better picture of the nerve or nerve types affected, as shown in Table 3.

Pain represents the most common symptom. Sharp, burning pain accompanied by paresthesia may be limited to a specific dermatome due to compression or incipient ischemia of sensory fibers. Compressed sensory fibers lead to a constellation of symptoms such as hyperesthesia, hypesthesia, hypalgesia, hyperalgesia, loss of two-point discrimination, or loss of vibratory sense. Compressed motor nerves create a diffuse deep pain that can be best localized to a muscle group or joint. However, nerve compression of any type can present with symptoms proximal and distal to the actual area involved. While the pain from tendinitis intensifies with motion and decreases with rest, the pain from a tunnel syndrome may actually be present at all times, worsen with motion, and wake one from sleep.

For example, carpal tunnel syndrome can masquerade as cervical spine or brachial plexus disease and vice versa, since their sensory and motor fields overlap. Therefore, physicians must be cautious in their approach to any neurological complaint. Motor nerve involvement can lead to weakness and atrophy secondary to denervation or disease due to pain. Assessing which muscle or muscles groups are affected helps differentiate which nerves are involved.

Since many nerves are mixed in nature, nerve compression varies in its presentation depending on whether sensory or motor nerve damage dominates. Vegetative symptoms can develop as autonomic fibers become involved. Disturbed sweating, one of the more noticeable symptoms, can be tested in the minhidrinic test. Decreased sweating is observed in the enervated area, allowing verification of the physical exam.

Tunnel syndromes require specific testing to determine the level of compression as well as the accuracy of the patient's presentation. Sensory symptoms and signs appear before motor signs; basing one's diagnosis and treatment upon the appearance of motor signs would place

TABLE 3
Examples of Syndromes Associated with Compression
of Different Nerve Types

Nerve type	General symptoms
Sensory	Loss of discrimination, sharp burning, vibratory sense, paresthesia, hyperthesias, hypalgesia, hyperesthesias, hyperalgesia, pain
Motor	Vague pain, blunt pain on appropriate muscle group pressure and us; night pain
Mixed	Combined and varying effects
Weakness	Muscle atrophy
Automatic	Vegetative disturbances; autonomic sweating/decreased

many patients in an unacceptable position. The length of the wait without any treatment might close off many conservative therapeutic options, since time under compression greatly decreases the chances for maximal nerve recovery. With prolonged nerve compression, impairment of motor strength and function become manifest. Typically, motor strength ranges from 0 to 5, as shown in Table 4. Understanding muscle-group innervation allows the physician to use the physical examination to delineate where compression occurs between the brain, the spinal cord, and the destination of the peripheral nerves. This understanding also allows the physician to find those patients with a true pathologic basis among groups of malingerers. Asymmetrical reflexes or a change in reflex strength indicates nerve root disease, as shown in Table 4.

While electrodiagnostic testing can indicate or confirm a diagnosis, the reliability and accuracy of electrodiagnostic testing depends on the tester as well as the nerve tested.[7,8] Therefore, the availability of these tests does not eliminate the need for a detailed history and physical. The contribution of electrodiagnostic testing is based on its ability to stimulate specific nerves in a constant and known fashion with an expected result. The failure of the nerve to respond in a timely and appropriate fashion is defined as pathologic. Patterns of response can indicate compression, division, degeneration, or regeneration at specific levels of the nerve's course. Evaluation of muscle response to direct nonneurogenic stimulation (galvanic, faradic steam) differentiates muscle from nerve pathology. Electromyography and nerve-conduction velocity studies help analyze the muscle's response to neural stimulation.

Electromyography records the muscle response to various neural stimuli. The muscle's intrinsic response can be judged from a resting state to a maximally stimulated state. While resting, few if any faasciculations should be appreciated. As nerve stimulation increases, more motor units should be recruited. Their recruitment comes in waves and will become superimposed during maximal stimulation. The patterns for voluntary action, denervation, compression, reinnervation, myopathy, and lower motor neuron disease are characteristic when fully developed. Therefore, testing may need to be repeated to clarify situations. Nerve-conduction velocity studies use maximal stimulation to assess the time between the stimulus and the motor response. The duration of the action potential and its amplitude can also be evaluated. By varying the stimulated point in the nerve's course, one may identify the site of the lesion. Motor and cutaneous afferent nerves may be tested in this manner. Each nerve has a characteristic conduction time and configuration; however, as noted above, one should not fully rely on these tests, since they require specialists. Furthermore, a normal or borderline normal electrodiagnostic battery does not exclude the existence of a tunnel syndrome.[9,10]

TABLE 4
Currently Used Muscle and Reflex Grading Systems

Grade	Motor	Reflex
0	Paralysis	Flaccid paralysis
1	Fasciculations	Hyporeflexia
2	Muscle contraction, no motion	Normal
3	Muscle motion with gravity eliminated	Hyperreflexia
4	Muscle action, weak	Hyperreflexia with clonous/spasticity
5	Maximal muscle action	

DIAGNOSIS

Diagnosis begins with a thorough history and physical exam. One should use technological tools to verify any hypothesis. However, the modern physical sometimes neglects the clinical examination and relies solely on laboratory tests, radiologic examinations, and electromyographyic studies for diagnosis. This approach places the cart before the horse. Wartenberg[11] wrote that if the laboratory examinations do not agree with the clinical findings, one should make the diagnosis based on the clinical findings. Thus, physicians should always reevaluate their hypothesis in the light of changes in their examinations or lab results and redirect their inquiries appropriately.

Understanding the etiology of a tunnel syndrome and the anatomy of the tunnel allows the physician to develop a hypothesis from the patient's history (Figures 1A and B). The history should direct one to an appropriate physical exam. If questions remain, then special tests may be ordered to differentiate among the possible disorders.[12-15] The history should elicit the patient's chief complaint whether it be pain, sensory disorders, or disturbances of mobility. Since descriptions can be confusing, one must explicitly determine what the patient means to say. Special attention must be paid to the following:

- When did the symptoms develop?
- Were they preceded by trauma, hospitalization, surgery, or immobilization?
- What is the actual complex of symptoms? (Care should be taken to differentiate pain from paresthesia and weakness, and temporary from permanent.)
- What areas are involved?
- Does anything relieve or aggravate the patient's symptoms?
- Has the patient been previously treated? How, and was treatment successful?
- What is the patient's profession and what physical tasks and mental stresses does it entail?
- What is the patient's dominant arm?
- What is the patient's general state of health (metabolic or hormonal disorders, developmental deformities, chronic contagious disease)?
- What is the patient's surgical and medical history?
- What medications does the patient take?

This approach should become routine to avoid missing any telltale signs.

Analysis of the history allows one to direct the patient's physical examination. This examination, in itself, should be methodological. First, one should inspect the skin and nails for dystrophic or atrophic changes. As dystrophic or infiltrative changes occur, the skin loses elasticity, splits, and becomes hyperkeratotic. This glossy skin proceeds to loss, blistering, ulcers, pigment changes in atrophoderma neuriticum. Hypertrichosis or hypotrichosis may also be a consequence of nerve injury. Nails may become thinner, break more easily, and have uneven

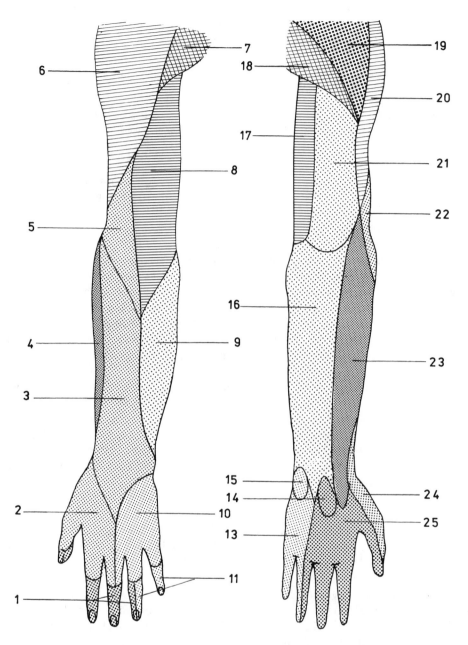

FIGURE 1A. This figure represents the dermatomes of the upper extremity. Having a working understanding of these dermatomes allows the physician to delineate the involved nerves.

1: Proper palmar digital nerves, median nerve; 2: superficial branch of the radial nerve; 3: posterior cutaneous nerve of the forearm, radial nerve; 4: lateral cutaneous nerve of the forearm, musculocutaneous nerve; 5: dorsal cutaneous nerve of the aarm, radial nerve; 6: axillary nerve, cutaneous branch; lower lateral cutaneous nerve of the arm (radial nerve); 7: cutaneous branches of the intercostal nerves; 8: medial cutaneous nerve of the arm; 9: medial cutaneous nerve of the forearm; 10: dorsal branch of the hand, ulnar nerve; 11: proper digital palmar nerves, ulnar nerve; 13: superficial branch of the radial nerve; 14: palmar branch of the median nerve; 15: palmar branch of the ulnar nerve; 16: medial cutaneous nerve of the forearm, palmar branch; 17: medial cutaneous nerve of the arm; 18: cutaneous branches of the intercostal nerves; 19: supraclavicular nerves; 20: axillary nerve, cutaneous branch; lower lateral cutaneous nerve of the arm, radial nerve; 21: medial cutaneous nerve of the arm; 22: lower lateral cutaneous nerve of the arm, radial nerve; 23: lateral cutaneous nerve of the forearm, musculocutaneous nerve; 24: superficial radial nerve; 25: palmar digital nerves, median nerve.

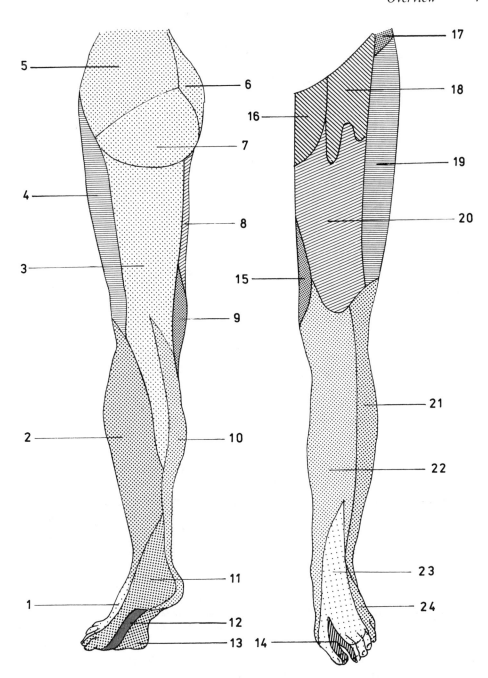

FIGURE 1B. This figure shows the dermatome pattern of the lower extremity.

1: Superficial peroneal nerve; 2: proximal section: lateral cutaneous nerve of the calf from the common peroneal nerve; distal section: superficial peroneal nerve; 3: posterior femoral cutaneous nerve; 4: lateral femoral cutaneous nerve; 5: superior (cranial) cluneal nerves; 6: inferior medial cluneal nerves; 7: inferior lateral cluneal nerves; 8: obtuator nerve. cutaneous branches; 9: medial cutaneous nerve of the thigh (from the femoral nerve); 10: saphenous nerve, medial cutaneous branches from the femoral nerve; 11: sural nerve; 12: lateral plantar nerve; 13: medial plantar nerve; 14: deep peroneal nerve; 15: obturator nerve, cutaneous branches; 16: combination of the ilioinguinal, genital, and genitofemoral nerves; 17: iliohypogastric nerve, lateral cutaneous branches; 18: genitofemoral nerve, femoral branch (also known as the lumboinguinal nerve); 19: lateral femoral cutaneous nerve; 20: intermediate and medial cutaneous nerves of the thigh (also known as anterior femoral nerve, cutaneous branches); 21: lateral cutaneous nerve of the calf, superficial peroneal nerve; 22: saphenous nerve, cutaneous branch; 23: superficial peroneal nerve; 24: sural nerve.

TABLE 5
Physical Signs

Physical area	Signs
Skin	Temperature
	Scars
	Dystrophic
	Hyperkeratotic
	Atrophic
	Glossy, red, hairless
	Sweating ability
Nails	Thickness
Muscles	Tone
	Bulk
	Strength
Skeleton	Deformities
	Anomalies
	Old fractures callus

surfaces; as in Alfod's syndrome, they may have white lines and nail-root elevation. These changes in skin and nails are rarely manifested to large degrees in tunnel syndromes, because partial innervation is usually maintained.

Nerve compression in the late stages leads to weakness and atrophy of the involved muscle groups. Inspection of a patient's overall symmetry, posture, scars, swelling, and static deformities, can raise or answer questions about his or her disease (Table 5). Paralysis of the radial or ulnar nerve will leave the upper extremities in characteristic positions, just as the patient with ilioinguinal nerve oppression can remind the physician of a person with appendicitis.

History and inspection target potential areas for palpation. Smooth skin that allows the hand to glide, decreased sweating, pain, and temperature differences found along the dermatome may be due to the involved nerve when compared to the patient's other side. To differentiate tunnel syndromes from ischemic diseases, peripheral pulses should be evaluated. While palpation can indicate painful or weak areas, the physician needs a detailed neurologic examination with objective tests.

Evaluation of pain requires a twofold approach — objective and subjective. Objective examination requires a cooperative patient and repetitive exams not only to follow the disease, but also to show consistency. One examines light touch, appreciation of temperature, two-point discrimination, vibrational sense, proprioception, pain, and graphesthesia. The standard neurological tests are not appropriate in children, mentally retarded persons, or people in extreme pain. One must remember that patients may exaggerate their problems. Therefore, with great patience, both the physician and the patient must experience thorough and repetitive exams, with accurate documentation of every time that the patient should respond.

Objective evaluation of pain is based on sweating in response to stimulation. Many investigators have developed tests, as listed in Table 6.[16-19] All require a reaction between sweat and indicators such as starch, chimisaum, and ninhidrin. One investigator has introduced the simple method of immersion of the affected area in 40°C water for 30 min.[20] While normal skin would wrinkle after prolonged exposure, skin in the dermatome of a compressed nerve remains smooth.

The aforementioned tests are clinically important as long as disturbances of sense do not coincide with disturbances of sweating. The autonomic nervous system controls the body's vegetative functions such as sweating. The hypothalamus processes differences between the

TABLE 6
Several Tests Available for Eliciting Nerve Compromise

Tested response	Test
Sensations	
Touch	Brush
Temperature	Hot/cold water in tubes
Pain	Needle, Tinel's
Vibration	Tuning fork
Graphasthesia	Coins, keys, writing
Two point	Calipers
Sweating	Minor (1928): iodine — starch
(sense of heat)	iodine on skin, then stress potato
	starch sweat caused a color change
	in the starch[17]
	Guttman (1931): Chinisarin on the
	skin, then rice-starch with a red
	color developing with sweat
	Moberg (1958): Ninhidrin soaked
	paper reacts with amino acid in
	sweat and when placed in an
	incubator becomes violet (amino
	acids: asparagine, gultaine,
	thiamine, valine, serence,
	methionine).

environmental temperature and the body's set point and reacts to maintain equilibrium by vasodilation and sweating to cool or by vasoconstriction to prevent heat loss. Peripheral control of sweating can be influenced by both pilocarpine and heat. Today computerized teleterography is available to diagnose tunnel syndromes.[21]

Radiographic studies have limited uses, since soft-tissue variations are the compressive agents in many tunnel syndromes. In the ambiguous cases, computed tomography (CT) and magnetic resonance imaging (MRI, NMR) will, with an increase in resolution and a refinement in application, be of use prior to surgical exploration.[22] Plain films can only reveal exostosis, callus, and anatomical anomalies. Special techniques like angiography can occasionally be used to assess the vascular contribution to a neurovascular compressive syndrome.

TREATMENT

Treatment of tunnel syndromes, whether conservative or surgical, must address the etiology causing nerve compression. While conservative measures of splinting and rest may relieve compression due to repetitive actions, they will be ineffective if the compression is caused by fracture callus, soft tissue compression, exostosis, or anatomical anomalies. Systemic or hormonal disease or changes may initiate or aggravate tunnel syndromes. Appropriate response to these causes may decrease the compression syndromes. Alleviating nerve compression becomes paramount, since time increases the risk of irreversible nerve injury.

Conservative measures consisting of immobilization, rest exercise, ultrasound, heat, massage, and anti-inflammatory medications may be tried where appropriate. These trials must be monitored to assess the patient's response. If symptoms worsen, one may try corticosteroid injections as the last conservative option prior to surgery. Steroid injections typically consist of a water-soluble, depot preparation introduced with a thin needle into the tunnel. The injection actually compounds the patient's complaints since it decreases the space remaining in the tunnel. The pain and stiffness decrease over two days as the inflammatory portion of the compression decreases. Injections may be tried several times; however, caution must be exercised, as repetitive steroid injections may damage tendons and joint surfaces. The physician and the patient must approach each conservative trial with a time limit in mind. If definitive therapy is postponed, the prognosis for nerve recovery worsens.

Surgical decompression remains the last resort when conservative therapy fails.[23-28] Semple and Cargil[29] demonstrated a 97% surgical success if decompression was performed with in six months of the onset of symptoms. Bilić and Pećina[1] felt that treatment depended on the status of the impaired nerve as assessed by clinical exam and specific tests.[30] Surgery allows direct visualization of the tunnel and the surrounding tissue. Failing that, some tunnel syndromes are treated by transposing the nerve. Neurolysis, tenosynovectomy, arthrodesis, or osteotomies may be required to increase the tunnel space within the tunnel.

REFERENCES

1. Kopell, H. P. and Thompson, W. A. L., *N. Engl. J. Med.*, 262, 56, 1960.
2. Lundborg, G., *J. Hand Surg.*, 4, 34, 1979.
3. Turek, S., *Orthopaedics: Principles and their Application*, 3rd ed., J. B. Lippincott, Philadelphia, 1977, pp. 407–447.
4. Bureau, H., Magalon, G., and Roffe, J. L., *J. Chir.* (Paris), 119, 739, 1982.
5. Horiuchi, Y., *J. Jpn. Orthop. Assoc.*, 57, 789, 1983.
6. Seddon, J. L., *J. Bone Joint Surg.*, 34, 386, 1952.
7. Jušic, A., Reumatizam (izvanredni broj IV) 1969, str. 141.
8. Wynn-Parry, C. B., Electrodiagnosis, in *The Hand*, Tubiana, R., Ed., W. B. Saunders, Philadelphia, 1981.
9. Lloyd, K. and Agarwal, A., *Br. Med. J.*, 3, 332, 1970.
10. Mumenthaler M. and Schliack, H., *Laisionen peripherer Nerven*, G. Theime, Stuttgart, 1965.
11. Wartenberg, R., *Neurologische Untersuchungsmethoden in der Sprechstunde*, G. Theime, Stuttgart, 1958.
12. Caffiniere, J. Y. and Theis, J. C., *Rev. Chir. Orthop.*, 70, 245, 1984.
13. Gilliat, R. W. and Wilson, T. G., *Lancet*, 2, 595, 1953.
14. Phalen, G. S., *J. Bone Joint Surg.*, 48A, 211, 1966.
15. Wormser, P., *Wortsch. Neurol. Physch.*, 18, 211, 1966.
16. Guttmann, L., *Fbl. Ges. Neurol. Psychiat.*, 135, 233, 1931.
17. Komar, J., *Alagut-szindromak*, Medician Könyvkiado, Budapest, 1977.
18. Moberg, E., *J. Bone Joint Surg.*, 40B, 454, 1958.
19. Tinel, J., *Presse Med.*, 23, 388, 1915.
20. O'Riain, S., *Br. Med. J.*, 3, 615, 1973.
21. Dumoulin, J., Clauses, T., and de Bisschop, G., *Electrodiagn. Ther.*, 18, 13, 1987.
22. Tackmann, W., Richter, H. P., and Stöhn, M., Kompressionssyndrome peripherer Nerven, Springer-Verlag, Berlin-Heidelberg, 1989.
23. Bora, F. W. and Osterman, L. A., *Clin. Orthop.*, 163, 20, 1982.
24. Dawson, D. M., Hallett, M., and Millender, L. H., *Entrapment Neuropathies*, Little, Brown, Boston, 1983.
25. Eversmann, W. W., Entrapment and compression neuropathies, in (*Operative Hand Surgery*) Green, D. P., Ed., Churchill Livingstone, New York, 1982.
26. Hurst, C. L., Badalamente, M. A., Paul, S., and Coyle, P. M., Peripheral nerve injuries and entrapments, in *Principles of Orthopaedic Practice*, Dee, R., Ed., McGraw-Hill, New York, 1989.
27. Souquet, R., Ed., *Syndromes Canalaires du Membre Superieur*, Expansion Scientifique Francaise, Paris, 1983.
28. Sunderland, S., *Nerves and Nerve Injuries*, 2nd ed., Churchill Livingstone, London, 1978.
29. Semple, J.C. and Cargill, A.O., *Lancet*, 3, 918, 1969.
30. Bilić, R. and Pećina, M., *Acta Orthop. Lugosl.*, 17, 191, 1986.

Part I

TUNNEL SYNDROMES IN THE UPPER EXTREMITIES

Media attention to nerve compression in the upper extremities has dramatically increased the number of patients presenting to physicians offices. While multiple etiologies for tunnel syndromes exist, recent literature has emphasized occupation-induced compression. Losing considerable productivity to tunnel syndromes, employers have sought to use pre-employment screening and job assessments by physicians and occupation therapists to decrease their vulnerability to workmen's compensation claims. Unfortunately, the long course of the nerves to the hands places them at risk in multiple locations and from various actions. This vulnerability complicates the physician's task of identifying the location and treating the compressive cause of the tunnel syndrome. Additionally the compression may be unrelated to the patient's occupation.

To sort through the confusion, a coordinated approach to diagnosis and treatment is recommended. Office practice should consistently look for the major causes and contributors to nerve compression in the history and physical. Protocols with both occupational and physical therapists should be pre-arranged and then tailored to the individual case. Investigative tests should be conducted based on the information gleaned from the history and physical. Repeat examinations including electromyographic studies or rheumatologic work-ups may be helpful before proceeding to more invasive modalities.

The list of potential etiologies for nerve compression in the upper extremity is long and may overlap. The physician must be able to isolate the primary etiology for the symptoms. Polyneuropathies and rheumatic disease can coexist causing localized exacerbations that are amenable to direct treatment. Treatment of ulnar or medial nerve compression in the forearm without regard to possible proximal compression (i.e. cervical spine disease) may leave the patient without relief despite adequate decompression. Relief of occupation-induced nerve compression without modification of the work environment may lead to only a temporary solution. Functional impairment cannot be excluded but should remain a diagnosis of exclusion.

Use of an ordered screening and testing process will help select those patients whose compressive symptoms represent true tunnel syndromes. The majority of these syndromes, when isolated, are amenable to either conservative or surgical modalities. Conservative treatment should be initiated first before considering surgical decompression. However, immediate surgical decompression may be necessary when confronted with signs and symptoms of prolonged nerve compression. Despite prompt and appropriate treatment, the outcome following nerve decompression may be varied. The following chapters address the screening, testing, and treatment of patients who present with complaints of nerve compression in the upper extremity.

THORACIC OUTLET SYNDROME

Upper extremity dysfunction may result from compression of the brachial plexus, the subclavian artery, or the subclavian vein before their division and separation. This area bears the name *thoracic outlet*.[1] Therefore, the syndrome of upper-limb pain, paresthesias, vascular insufficiency, and motor dysfunction secondary to compression bears the name *thoracic outlet syndrome*. Its clinical presentation varies depending on where and which neurovascular structures are compressed. The term was first used in 1956 by Peet et al.[2] Careful review of the literature reveals descriptions of similar syndromes: the anterior scalene syndrome by Adson and Coffey[3] in 1927; the costoclavicular syndrome by Falconer and Wedell[4] in 1943, and hyperabduction syndrome by Wright[5] in 1945. The thoracic outlet syndrome has been extensively investigated to help accurately diagnose, evaluate etiologies, and expediently treat patients presenting with vague symptoms. The present standard is dependent not only on those authors noted in this chapter, but also on all those whose efforts have yielded this body of knowledge.

For didactic reasons, this chapter will present the thoracic outlet syndrome in separate syndromes as it was chronologically described in medical literature.

ANTERIOR SCALENE SYNDROME

The brachial plexus and the subclavian artery can be compressed as they pass between the anterior and medial scalene muscles and the first rib, yielding a characteristic neurovascular syndrome, the anterior scalene syndrome.

All three scalene muscles originate from the transverse processes of the cervical vertebrae and insert on the first and second ribs. The anterior and medial scalene muscles insert on the respective tubercles on the first rib, sandwiching the subclavian artery into a sulcus (Figure 1). The posterior scalenus muscle is fixed to the second rib. A variable scalenus minimus muscle may exist and insert between the anterior and medial scalenus muscles. The scalene muscles raise the first and second rib during inspiration. Unilateral contraction inclines the head to the side of action and turns the face to the opposite side. Bilateral contraction flexes the cervical spine. The anterior and medial scalene muscles form one side of the scalene foramen, with the sternocleidomastoid muscle and the first rib forming the other sides. Bounded by the anterior scalene muscle, the first rib, and the medial scalene muscle, the posterior scalene foramen admits the brachial plexus and the subclavian artery to the costoclavicular space. The posterior foramen can range from 0.4 to 3.5 cm in width.[6]

The subclavian artery bends over and tracts through a sulcus in the first rib. Composed of nerve roots from C5 to C8 and T1, the brachial plexus represents the innervation of the entire upper extremity and lies tautly stretched and without bony protection in this region.

Neurovascular compression can occur when disease or anatomical variations narrow a tight foramen. In the development of the anterior scalenus syndrome, some anatomical variations are very important.[7] They shall be described among the causes producing the syndrome.

ETIOLOGY

The anterior scalene syndrome has many similarities with the costoclavicular syndrome, also known as the syndrome of the cervical rib. Willshire[8] in 1860 and Gruber[9] in 1869 described the syndrome of the cervical rib. Murphy[10] described the neurovascular changes due to compression between the cervical rib and anterior scalenus muscle. Naffziger and Grant[11] and Ochsner, Gage, and Debakey[12] have published cases where the anterior scalenus muscle alone,

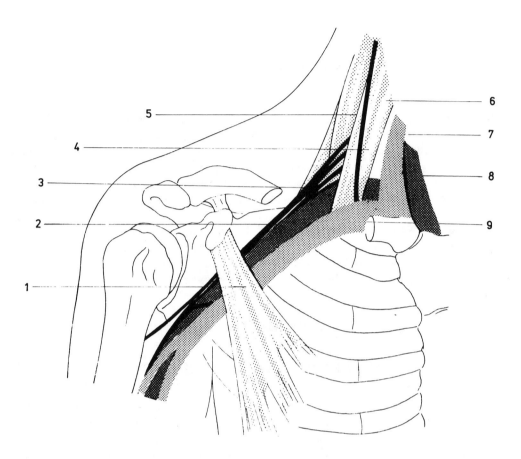

FIGURE 1.   This figure illustrates the region of the thoracic outlet where the brachial plexus lies exposed to bony, muscular, vascular, neoplastic, and traumatic compression.
1: Pectoralis minor muscle; 2: subclavian artery; 3: brachial plexus; 4: anterior scalene muscle; 5: phrenic nerve; 6: anterior scalene muscle; 7: internal jugular vein; 8: common carotid artery; 9: subclavian vein.

without the existence of the cervical rib, is responsible for the compression of the neurovascular bundle with corresponding clinical symptoms. Komar[13] summarized literature reviews of anterior scalenus syndromes.

Under normal circumstances, there is enough room in the posterior scalene foramen for the brachial plexus and the subclavian artery. However, many anatomical variations and consequences of changes in the functional anatomy of the shoulder and upper extremity can cause the development of the clinical symptoms.[14] Lord and Rosati[9] stress that many embryological, anatomical, and physiological factors create a disposition for development of compression in the posterior scalene foramen. According to these authors, the roots of the brachial plexus and the subclavian artery are bent under tension over the first rib, due to the change from the posture of a quadrupe to the erect posture in man.

A quadruped's thorax has its largest diameter in the anterior posterior dimension. A man's thorax has its largest diameter in the laterolateral dimension. The asymmetry of the thorax places man's nerves and arteries in a position of tension.[15] Poor posture, prolonged work above one's head, prolonged wearing of a knapsack, or advanced age may produce a lowered or anteriorly rotated shoulder and further increase the distance the nerves and vessels must travel.[16-20] In adult women, the shoulder has a lower position in relation to the thorax than in men. Carrying heavy burdens on one's arms produces cervicobrachial destination that, when combined with increased respiratory excursion due to work, results in tension over the scalene foramen. The asymmetry of the foramen contributes to the unfavorable situation. The presence of a cervical rib or scalenus minumus muscle plays a role by either raising the floor of the foramen or narrowing the foramen in the anteroposterior dimension. While this etiology was the first to be noted, Swank and Simeone[21] and more recently, Frankel and Hirata[22] stress the importance of scalenus muscle hypertrophy in narrowing the foramen. Chronic vibrating trauma has also been implicated.[23,24] A cervical rib is, however, not the only reason for development of the syndrome.[25] The insertions of the anterior and medial scalene muscles on the first rib may approach each other, thereby narrowing the sulcus. Fibrous bands may connect the anterior and posterior scalene muscles producing a sling that elevates the brachial plexus and the subclavian artery over the first rib.[9] Some authors believe that even an unusually strong contraction of the anterior scalene muscle can profoundly elevate the first rib further narrowing the foramen. However, Telford and Mottershead[26] found the first rib to still be a problem despite sectioning of the anterior scalene muscle in a series of hundreds of patients.

The vascular symptoms in the anterior scalene syndrome occur from tension of the artery or vein over the first rib.[27,28] Distal to the area of arterial compression or occlusion,[29] one may find a post-stenotic dilation. Vegetative nerve fibers are compressed at the same time as the neurovascular bundle.[23,24]

CLINICAL SYMPTOMS AND SIGNS

The neurovascular symptomatology depends upon the frequency, duration, and degree of compression of the subclavian artery and the brachial plexus. The lower roots of the brachial plexus (C8-T1) are at higher risk of compression than the higher roots, due to their location in the plexus. The symptoms generally include pain in the fingers, hand, forearm, arm, and even the shoulder, with paresthesias and hyperesthesias especially in the eight cervical and first thoracic nerve root dermatomes. Numbness appears more often in the fingers, hand, and forearm. Depending upon the degree of arterial compression, ischemic symptoms of numbness, cold, weakness, and skin-color changes appear. Gangrene and ulcerations of the fingers may develop in severe cases. Ischemic pain can closely approximate pain from nerve compression. Weakened grip and impaired finger function may be present. According to Komar,[13] the symptoms can be arranged in four groups: symptoms due to neurological dysfunction; symptoms due to vascular compression; symptoms due to different body postures; and symptoms due to functional and anatomical changes of the scalene foramen.

Neurological symptoms correspond to the compression of the inferior part of the brachial plexus (C8, T1), resulting in paresis and hypotrophy of the hypothenar and interossei muscles. Vascular symptoms are manifested as intermittent ischemic crises similar to Raynaud's phenomenon. Distal to the site of arterial compression can lie an aneurysm where thrombi may develop. Freed emboli can obliterate one of the terminal finger arteries, an occurrence that is followed by severe pain. Adson's sign represents a diagnostic test to elicit symptoms based on body posture. The sign utilizes movements that stretch the anterior and medial scalene muscles and create the possibility of neurovascular compression in the region of the first rib. The examiner evaluates the strength of the radial pulse in the hanging arm as the patient inspires deeply, extends the neck, and turns the head in both directions. Since the pulse may weaken or disappear in normal subjects, one must also examine other signs and perform other tests such as arteriography before proceeding to surgery. Arteriography, ultrasound, or auscultation may allow detection of subclavian artery compression during an Adson's test. When normal posture is regained, the pulse of a normal person with a positive Adson's test will return much quicker than that of a person with the anterior scalene syndrome.[13] French investigators describe an additional test, the *signe des plateau*. The arm is abducted and placed parallel to the ground with the palm up. In contrast to the situation when the patient's arm is supported in this position, the radial pulse disappears when resistance is applied to the arm. Rather than depend on palpation, oscillography may be used. The presence of a cervical rib may be seen on plain radiographs.

Hypertrophied and taut anterior scalenus muscles and cervical ribs may be palpated in the supraclavicular region. While more than one test is available, none are absolute, thus creating an atmosphere for initially trying conservative therapy.

TREATMENT

Treatment depends on the degree of subjective symptoms and objective signs. With mild symptoms or incomplete signs, conservative therapy should be applied even in cases with an identifiable cervical rib. Conservative treatment includes physical therapy, immobilization, ultrasound, and corticosteroid injections. Physical therapy seeks to increase tone in the shoulder muscles to decrease the tone in the cervical musculature. Immobilization is combined with physical therapy to keep the shoulder from continuing to drag between therapy sessions. If symptoms become severe, surgical decompression consisting of scalenotomy or cervical rib resection[32] has a 50% success rate.[33] Some authors advise combining scalenotomy, sympathectomy, and even first-rib resection.[34] To this day, neither the best surgical procedure nor the best time for intervention has been found.[1,35]

COSTOCLAVICULAR SYNDROME

Costoclavicular syndrome occurs with compression of the subclavian artery, subclavian vein, and brachial plexus as they pass between the clavicle and the first rib. Falconer and Weddell[4] describe this syndrome as separate from the anterior scalene syndrome due to the vascular involvement.

ANATOMY

The costoclavicular space, triangular in shape, connects the cervical spine with the upper extremity, and thus also bears the name *canalis cervicoaxillris*. The boundaries of this space are the following: anteriorly, the medial third of the clavicle and the subclavius muscle; posterolaterally, the upper margin of the scapula; and posteromedially, the anterior third of the first rib and the insertions of the anterior and medial scalene muscles (Figure 2). The neurovascular bundle runs in the medial angle of this triangle. The subclavian vein lies medially in front of the anterior scalenus muscle's insertion on the first rib and deep to the costoclavicular ligament and thickening of the clavipectoral fascia, which extends from the coracoid process to the first rib (costocoracoid ligament). The subclavian artery briefly enters this space via the posterior scalene foramen to lie lateral to the subclavian vein. Passing between the anterior and medial scalenus muscles, the brachial plexus joins the vascular bundle in the costoclavicular space.

ETIOLOGY

When the costoclavicular space becomes narrowed by disease or dynamic compression, the neuromusucular structures are compromised.[36-38] Roos and Owens[39] described congenital anomalies associated with thoracic outlet syndrome. Functional or dynamic anatomy predominates as an etiology for clinical disease.[40] Three reactions narrow the space: raising one's arm rotates the clavicle posteriorly into the space; displacing one's shoulder posteriorly and interiorly rotates the clavicle posteriorly; and inhaling deeply raises the first rib into the space, since the clavicle does not rise with inspiration.

CLINICAL SYMPTOMS AND SIGNS

Patients with costoclavicular syndrome present similar subjective complaints as those with the anterior scalenus syndrome. While the neurological complaints of pain, paresthesia, and hyperesthesia dominate in the anterior scalenus syndrome, vascular symptoms dominate in the costoclavicular syndrome.[41] Vein compression leads to the temporary or permanent edema.

Clinical examination relies on radial artery pulse evaluation when the patient thrusts the chest forward and pulls the shoulders posteriorly and interiorly. Typically the pulse weakens or

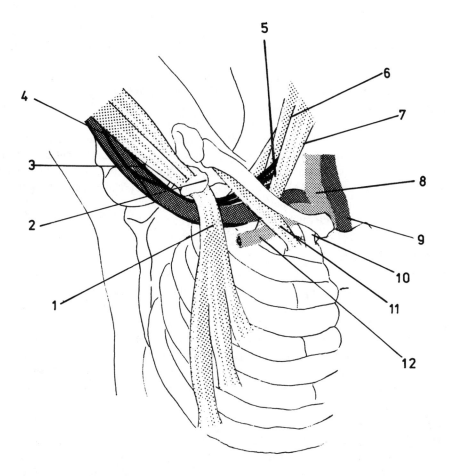

FIGURE 2.   Dynamic anatomical variations of tunnels have been postulated as possible etiologies for various tunnel syndromes. This figure shows dynamic compression of the brachial plexus in the thoracic outlet.

1: Pectoralis minor muscle; 2: coracoid process; 3: median nerve; 4: subclavian artery; 5: brachial plexus; 6: medial scalene muscle; 7: anterior scalene muscle; 8: internal jugular vein; 9: common carotid artery; 10: costoclavicular ligament; 11: subclavious muscle; 12: subclavian vein.

disappears. Electric measurement through oscilloscope can verify these changes. However, pulse damping can occur in controls.[42] Komar[13] recommended arteriography to evaluate the changes in flow between positions. Venography and venous pressure measurements have been proposed to aid in evaluation.

TREATMENT

Conservative therapy consisting of physical therapy and temporary immobilization may be tried. If the etiology can be identified, surgical removal of the agent is warranted, whether it be a pseudoarthrosis of the clavicle, an exuberant callus, or an impinging first rib.

HYPERABDUCTION SYNDROME

In repetitive or prolonged hyperabduction of the arm, the neurovascular bundle in the axilla can be stretched under the pectoralis minor tendon and the coracoid process, resulting in symptoms of neurovascular compression. This collection of symptoms, known as the hyperabduction syndrome, was first described by Wright in 1945.[5]

ANATOMY

Leaving the costoclavicular space, the three cords of the brachial plexus, the subclavian artery, and the subclavian vein pass under the insertion of the pectoralis minor muscle on the coracoid process. As this neurovascular bundle enters the axillary fossa, the artery and vein become known as the axillary artery and the axillary vein (Figures 1 and 2). As the upper extremity is abducted to 180°, the neurovascular bundle is stretched around a fulcrum consisting of the tendon of the pectoralis minor, the coracoid process, and the humeral head. The bundle almost reaches an angle of 90° around the fulcrum. Unfortunately, the neurovascular bundle's course remains fixed, allowing relatively no motion of the bundle. The bundle can only compensate by compression at the fulcrum and tension along its components. Abduction of the arm produces a 30° elevation and a 35° posterior displacement of the clavicle, thereby narrowing the costoclavicular tunnel. The tunnel's anterior wall, consisting also of the pectoralis minor muscle, the subclavius muscle, and the costoclavicular ligament (the thickening of the clavipectoral fascia), is stretched and brought posteriorly further, pushing the neurovascular bundle against the fulcrum.

ETIOLOGY

Wright[5] describes two critical anatomical points where compression of the neurovascular bundle may occur with the arm in hyperabduction: the first, while passing through the costoclavicular tunnel or slit; and the second, while passing under the pectoralis minor tendon at its insertion on the coracoid process. During abduction of the arm, the fixed neurovascular bundle can be compressed by the tendon of the pectoralis minor muscle as well as by the humeral head.[43] The characteristic position described is 180° of shoulder abducted and elbow flexion. This position commonly occurs during sleep or in professionals like electricians, painters, bricklayers, or masons.

CLINICAL SYMPTOMS AND SIGNS

Pain, paresthesia, and numbness develop first in the fingers and later in the hand. In some patients, transitory ischemia and edema develop. These symptoms may resemble Raynaud's disease, which Beyer and Wright[44] described as being present in 38% of patients with hyperabduction syndrome. Neurological symptoms are usually absent in hyperabduction syndrome, because as paresthesia and pain develop, the patients correct their arm position, so that the nerve compression only lasts a short time. If the arm is abducted to 180° in patients with hyperabduction syndrome, the subjective symptoms can increase, while the radial artery pulse may weaken or disappear. However just as tests for the anterior scalene syndrome or the costoclavicular syndrome can be positive in a normal position, the same results can be found when testing for the hyperabduction syndrome. Additionally, while the Adson's test may be positive, Youman and Smiley[45] described the occurrence of thoracic Outlet syndrome with negative Adson's and hyperabduction maneuvers.

Strauer and Rastan[46] proposed venography, arteriography, and intra-arterial pressure measurements to accurately assess variations in an arm's vascular status with position.

TREATMENT

Treatment consists of avoiding hyperabduction. This may necessitate changes in one's workplace or habits. Operative therapy is infrequently indicated and consists in sectioning of the pectoralis minor tendon.

REFERENCES

1. Narakas, A., Bonnard, C., and Egloff, D. V., *Ann. Chir. Main,* 5, 195, 1986.
2. Peet, R. M., Hendricksen, J. D., Gunderson, T. P., and Martin, G. M., *Mayo Clin. Proc.,* 31, 281, 1956.
3. Adson, A. W. and Coffey, J. R., *Ann. Surg.,* 85, 839, 1927.
4. Falconer, M. A. and Weddell, G., *Lancet,* 2, 539, 1943.
5. Wright, I. S., *Am. Heart J.,* 29, 1, 1945.
6. Reisinger, G. and Türk, G., *Münch. Med. Wochenschr.,* 111, 2334, 1969.
7. McCleery, R. S., Kesterson, J. E., Kirtly, J. A., et al., *Ann. Surg.,* 133, 588, 1951.
8. Wilshire, W. H., *Lancet,* 2, 633, 1860.
9. Lord, W. J. and Rosati, M. L., *Clinical Symposia* (Ciba-Geigy), 23, 2, 1971.
10. Murphy, J. B., *Ann. Surg.,* 41, 399, 1905.
11. Naffziger, H. C. and Grant, W. T., *Surg. Gynecol. Obstet.,* 67, 722, 1938.
12. Ochsner, A., Gage, M., and De Bakey, M., *Am. J. Surg.,* 28, 669, 1935.
13. Komar, J., *Alagut-szindromak,* Medicina Könyvkiado, Budapest, 1977.
14. Thomas, G. I., Jones, T. W., Stavney, L. S., and Manhas, D. R., *Am. J. Surg.,* 145, 589, 1983.
15. Walshe, F., Disease of the nervous system, 10th ed., Livingstone, Edinbourgh, 1963.
16. Bom, F., *Acta Psychiatr. Scand.,* 28, 1, 1953.
17. Bourrel, P., Blanc, J. F., and Maistre, B., *Marseille Chir.,* 20, 375, 1970.
18. Bourrel, P. and Maistre, B., Syndrome du hile du membre supérieur, in *Syndromes Canalaires du Membre Supérieur,* Souquet, R., Ed., Expansion Scientifique Francaise, Paris, 1983.
19. Daube, J. R., *JAMA,* 208, 13, 1969.
20. Kremer, R. M. and Ahlquist, R. E., *Am. J. Surg.,* 130, 612, 1975.
21. Swank, R. L. and Siomeone, F. A., *Arch. Neurol. Psych.,* 51, 432, 1944.
22. Frankel, S. A. and Hirata, I., *JAMA,* 215, 1976, 1971.
23. Owens, J. C., Blaney, L. F., and Roos, D. B., *Bull. Soc. Int. Chir.,* 25, 547, 1966.
24. Kakosy, T. and Horvath, F., *Z. Orthop.,* 106, 98, 1969.
25. Brannon, E. W., *J. Bone Joint Surg.,* 45, A977, 1963.
26. Telford, F. D. and Mottershead, S., *J. Bone Joint Surg.,* 30B, 249, 1948.
27. Graber, S., as cited in Stammer, F. A. R., *Lancet,* 1, 603, 1950.
28. Lowenstein, P. S., *JAMA,* 82, 854, 1924.
29. Rob, C. G. and Standeven, A., *Br. Med. J.,* 2, 709, 1958.
30. Adson, A. W., *Surg. Gynecol. Obstet.,* 85, 687, 1947.
31. Adson, A. W., *J. Int. Coll. Surg.,* 16, 546, 1951.
32. Raaf, J., *JAMA,* 157, 219, 1955.
33. Bruis, 1976.
34. Roos, D. B., *Surgery,* 92, 1007, 1982.
35. Sedel, L. and Ducloyer, Ph., *Rev. Rhum. Mal. Osteoartic,* 55, 113, 1988.
36. Cliffton, E. E., *Arch. Surg.,* 55, 732, 1947.
37. Dorazio, R. A. and Ezzet, F., *Am. J. Surg.,* 138, 246, 1979.
38. Heyden, B. and Vollmar, J., *J. Cardiovasc. Surg.,* 20, 531, 1979.
39. Roos, D. B. and Owens, J. C., *Arch. Surg.,* 93, 71, 1966.
40. Winsor, T. and Brow, R., *JAMA,* 196, 109, 1966.
41. Klanfar, Z., Loverenic, M., Jakovac, I., Despot, I., and Kovac, D., *Lijec. Vjesn.,* 110, 361, 1988.
42. Gergouldis, R. and Barnes, R. W., *Angiology,* 31, 538, 1980.
43. Fields, W. S., Lemak, N. A., and Ben-Menachem, Y., *Am. J. Neuroradiol.,* 7, 73, 1986.
44. Beyer, J. A. and Wright, I. S., *Circulation,* 4, 161, 1951.
45. Youmans, C. R. and Smiley, R. H., *Vasc. Surg.,* 14, 318, 1980.
46. Strauer, B. E. and Rastan, H., *Dtsch. Med. Wochenschr.,* 97, 1335, 1975.

SCAPULOCOSTAL SYNDROME

GENERAL

In the shoulder region, especially along the medial border of the scapula, pain may develop and radiate into the neck, the brachium, and eventually the thorax, where it can be mistaken for angina pectoralis. Paresthesia and subjective weakness may complete the symptoms of this syndrome. Michele et al.[1] in 1950 coined the term *scapulocostal syndrome;* Moseley[2] and Steindler and Marxer[3] in the 1940s described symptoms inherent to it.

ANATOMY

The scapula, the focal point for upper-extremity function, serves as the origin or insertion of no less than 15 muscles and 6 ligaments, which allows man the intricate as well as general functions of the arm. The scapula sits with its superior and its inferior angle level with the second and seventh thoracic vertebrae, respectively. Underneath lie the posterior rami of thoracic nerves two through seven, the erector spinae muscles (spinalis, longissimus, iliocostalis), the serratus posterior and superior muscles, and the thoracolumbar fascia. The levator scapulae, major and minor rhomboid, trapezius, serratus anterior, and pectoralis minor muscles all insert on portions of the scapula. These muscles, with the assistance of several ligaments, suspend the scapula and position it in space to allow function. The shoulder gives rise to the deltoid, teres minor and major, biceps, coracobrachialis, supraspinatus, infraspinatus, subscapularis, and triceps muscles. These muscles suspend the upper extremity from the nearly vertical glenohumeral joint with the assistance of the glenohumeral and coracohumeral ligaments. The axillary nerve runs in close proximity to the glenohumeral joint. While all these muscles and ligaments must function simultaneously to allow mobility, dysfunction of even one can hamper activity and possibly set up a cycle of pain.

ETIOLOGY

The exact etiology of the scapulocostal syndrome remains unknown, although many hypotheses exist. Russek[4] holds, as a major determinate, poor posture resulting from one of the following sources: idiopathic poor posture; anatomical or functional deformity secondary to neck or shoulder injury; and static anatomic predilection. Poor posture places the scapula at an unfavorable angle with the chest wall, a situation that may produce dysfunction or pain. Some professions, such as stenographer, truck driver, and even surgeon, place the individual into contorted positions. Michele et al.[1] and McGovney[5] explain the syndrome in light of a segmental reflex mechanism. They propose that nerves from the cervical roots pass through the prevertebral fascia and may be irritated by muscular spasm or fibromyositis. Suspended from and lying in close proximity to the cervical spine, the scapula and its associated musculature receive segmental irritations. Scapulocostral syndrome can develop secondary to trauma or prolonged immobilization, boyh of which weaken the muscular girdle. The shoulder adjusts with compensatory measures, which over time lead to dysfunctional motion. Russek[4] identified shoulder subluxation, humeral fractures, and rotator cuff injuries as predisposing factors to scapulocostal syndrome development. Shull[6] believes the syndrome to be the result of various pathological factors.

CLINICAL SYMPTOMS AND SIGNS

In light of the proposed etiologies, which center on the cervical spine and the shoulder girdle, one can understand that patients will present with pain in the neck, upper arm, and chest. The pain and its pattern of radiation can be explained by shoulder-girdle spasm. Pain tends to culminate towards evening, but it is not aggravated by arm or shoulder motion. While patients may complain of paresthesia or muscle weakness, examination reveals no sensory deficit nor motor paralysis or atrophy. Physical examination may reveal a localized point on the medial scapular border where pressure reproduces the patient's pain.[7] Russek[4] describes another sign: scapular elevation off the chest wall with a forward stretch.

TREATMENT

Treatment should address the basis of the scapulocostal syndrome; therefore, the circular pattern of spasm and pain may be treated with infiltration of trigger zones with anesthetic followed by physical therapy to decrease spasm. Shull[6] had good results from cooling the trigger zones. Postures may be modified by physical therapy or surgical correction of gross deformity.

REFERENCES

1. Michele, A. A., Davies, J. J., Krueger, F. J., and Lichter, J. M., *N.Y. State J. Med.,* 50, 1353, 1950.
2. Moseley, H. F., *Shoulder Lesions,* C. C. Thomas, Springfield, MA, 1945.
3. Steindler, A. L. and Marxer, J. L., *The Traumatic Deformities and Disabilities of the Upper Extremity,* C. C. Thomas, Springfield, MA, 1946.
4. Russek, A. S., *JAMA,* 150, 25, 1952.
5. McGovney, R. B., *Clin. Orthop.,* 8, 191, 1956.
6. Shull, J. R., *St. Med. J.,* 62, 956, 1969.
7. Komar, J., *Alagut-szindromak,* Medicina-Könyvkiado, Budapest, 1977.

SUPRASCAPULAR NERVE SYNDROME
(INCISURA SCAPULAE SYNDROME)

The suprascapular nerve courses through the incisura scapulae bounded by the sharp margins of the scapula and the transverse scapular ligament. Compression or stretching of the nerve results in the development of suprascapular nerve syndrome, as first described by Andre Thomas in 1936.[1]

ANATOMY

Originating from either the C5 or C6 nerve roots or the upper trunk of the brachial plexus, the suprascapular nerve passes in a superoposterior fashion through the supraclavicular fossa and then the scapular notch to reach the supraspinatus fossa. The transverse scapular ligament forms a strong sometimes ossified bridge over the notch and nerve. The suprascapular vessels cross above the ligament rather than running with the nerve through the notch. The notch can occasionally be replaced by a foramen, the foramen scapulae. This foramen can become stenotic and squeeze the nerve. Occassionally, veins or even a branch of the suprascapular artery may run through the notch or foramen. At the incisura scapulae, the suprascapular nerve sends branches to the supraspinatus muscle, the acromioclavicular joint and bursa, and the subacromial bursa. The shoulder joint receives branches from the bursa branches and the nerve itself.

Accompanied by vessels in the supraspinatus fossa, the nerve passes through the muscle, sending at least one branch to the muscle. The neurovascular bundle bends around the base of the scapular spine and enters the infraspinatus fossa. In approximately 30% of individuals, the nerve may make a 90° turn, run along the scapular spine in the fossa, and give off three branches (Figure 1). To complicate matters, a connective tissue band, the ligamentum spinoglenoidale, may exist in up to 50% of people, creating a second fibro-osseus opening for the nerve to transverse. The suprascapular nerve stretches as the scapula moves. Since the nerve passes around rigid structures, functional anatomy plays a major role in understanding compression. Strong and sudden motions, including protraction and abduction, pull the nerve against the medial wall of the scapular notch or the ligament. External humeral rotation pulls the nerve against the lateral margin of the notch as the infraspinatus muscle interferes with its freedom of motion. Elevation and rotation of the arm also places a stretch on the nerve.

ETIOLOGY

As the scapula moves over the rib cage to optimize its position in function, the suprascapular nerve must adapt or be injured by repetitive stretches. Any disease process that limits its flexibilty or interferes with its route will increase its risk of damage. Few other nerves are placed in such a position of constant motion requiring an unobstructed course. Fractures of the scapula, including the scapular foramen,[2] may cause direct nerve compression. Bony or soft tissue injuries in the shoulder can alter the muscle tensions and bony relations enough to distort the nerve's course and lead to compression at the foramen. Chronic mechanical irritation due to repetitive nerve compression from stretching can occur, especially in individuals who work above their heads or place their arms into extremes of abduction and external rotation. Although sleeping with one's arms extended above the head may produce symptoms, the syndrome has been more frequently described in painters, electricians, volleyball and tennis players, weight lifters, and boxers. Ferretti et al.[3] described 12 volleyball players with asymptomatic isolated paralysis of the infraspinatus muscle on their dominant side. These findings were attributed to the repeated stress of the cocking of the arm and follow-through when the athlete serves. Shoulder pain from a variety of etiologies[4] creates a viscous circle of muscle decompensation

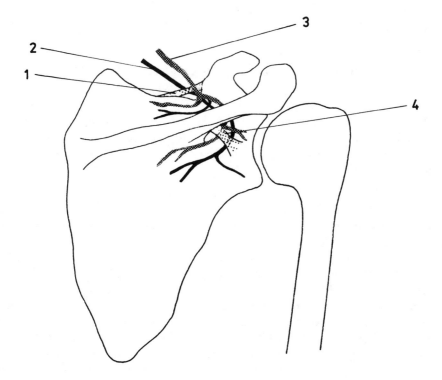

FIGURE 1.   This figure illustrates the suprascapular notch and the pertinent anatomical relationships of the scapula and ligament to the neurovascular bundle.
1: Transverse scapular ligament; 2: superscapular nerve; 3: superscapular artery; 4: spinoglenoid
ligament

and altered scapular function that places the suprascapular nerve at risk for compression at the
notch (Figure 1).

CLINICAL FINDINGS

Diagnosis of the syndrome of the suprascapular nerve remains difficult and many times
unrecognized because the predominant symptom of pain is common to many other disorders.
Shoulder pain can come from such varied etiologies such as rotator cuff tears, cervical spine
disease, scapulocostale syndrome, painful atrophy of shoulder muscles (Parsonage-Turner's
syndrome), and musculoskeletal strain; therefore, the physician must continuously reevaluate
his differential diagnosis. Many authors have provided information on this disease.[3-24] However,
the pain does not localize to a specific portion of the shoulder. The pain can range from deep and
blunt to sharp with radiation down the radial nerve's distribution, depending upon the shoulder
motion eliciting the pain. The suprascapular and radial nerve have common root origins;
therefore, painful stimulation may wash over at times. Pain is more commonly appreciated over
the posterior portion of the shoulder along the border of the trapezius muscle with pain
worsening at night. Once damaged, stretching of the nerve during daily activities that are as
simple as shaving or combing one's hair may aggravate the pain.

Clinical examination reveals a painful spot along the lateral third of the upper border of the
trapezius muscle over the scapular notch. The remainder of the shoulder may not be painful to
pressure. Active and passive range of motion exercises will create tension and reproduce the
patient's pain. The crossed abduction test seeks to elicit the patient's pain in the following way:
place the arm of the painful side on the healthy shoulder, then pull the elbow along the horizontal
towards the healthy shoulder.[14] This will accentuate the nerve's compression in the scapula's

notch. Within 3 to 4 months from the onset of pain, motor symptoms like supraspinatus and infraspinatus hypotrophy may develop. Compensation by other muscles in the shoulder girdle cover the loss of strength in abduction and rotation. Esslen et al.[9] found teres minor hypertrophy. Pain in the acromioclavicular joint and reduced sensitivity to vibration in the same region complete the clinical picture of the syndrome. Difficult to access for electrodiagnostic studies, the suprascapular nerve, when compressed, produces electromyographic changes of prolonged latency to the infraspinatus and supraspinatus muscles.

TREATMENT

Treatment must start with avoidance of all activities that place the nerve under stretch. Infiltration of the scapular notch with anesthetics and corticosteroids using fluoroscopic guidance can be diagnostic as well as therapeutic. Failure to respond to conservative approaches mandates surgical release of the transverse scapular ligament,[17,19,24] opening of the scapular foramen if present, and possibly neurolysis.

REFERENCES

1. Thomas, A., *Press Med.,* 44, 1283, 1936.
2. Edelan, H. G. and Zachrisson, B. E., *Acta Orthop. Scand.,* 46, 758, 1975.
3. Ferretti, A., Cerullo, G., and Russo, G., *J. Bone Joint Surg.,* 69A, 260, 1987.
4. Komar, J., *Orv. Hetil.,* 116, 1332, 1975.
5. Aiello, I., Serra, G., Traince, G. C., and Tognoli, V., *Ann Neurol.,* 12, 314, 1982.
6. Augustin, P., Verdun, L., and Samson, M., *Rev. Neurol.,* 132, 219, 1976.
7. Bauer, B. and Vogelsang, H., *Mschr. Unfalheilk,* 65, 461, 1962.
8. Domljan, Z., *Lijec. Vjesn.,* 91, 959, 1969.
9. Esslen, E., Falcshmann, H., Bishoff, A., Regli, F., and Ricklin, P., *Nervenarzt,* 38, 311, 1967.
10. Fassina, A., *Ortop. Reumat.,* 97, 255, 1984.
11. Ganzhorn, R. W., Hocker, J. T., Horowitz, M. I., and Switzer, H. E., *J. Bone Joint Surg.,* 63A, 492, 1981.
12. Garcia, G. and McGueen, D., *J. Bone Joint Surg.,* 63, 491, 1981.
13. Kaspi, A., Yanai, J., Pick, C. G., and Mann, G., *Int. Orthopaed.,* 12, 273, 1988.
14. Kopell, H. P. and Thompson, W. A. L., *N. Engl. J. Med.,* 260, 1261, 1959.
15. Mestdagh, H., Drizenko, A., and Ghesten, Ph., *Anatomia clinica,* 3, 67, 1981.
16. Mumenthaler, M. and Schliack, H., *Läsionen peripherer Nerven,* G. Thieme, Stuttgart, 1965.
17. Murray, J. W. G., *Orthop. Rev.,* 3, 33, 1974.
18. Picot, Cl., *Rhumatologie,* 21, 367, 1969.
19. Rask, M. R., *Clin. Orthop.,* 123, 73, 1978.
20. Schilf, E., *Nervenartz,* 23, 306, 1953.
21. Serre, S., *Rev. Rhum. Mal. Osteoartic.,* 5, 231, 1966.
22. Wells, R., *Suprascapular Nerve Entrapment in Injuries of the Throwing Arm,* W. B. Saunders, Philadelphia, 1985, 173–175.
23. Zoltan, J. D., *J. Trauma,* 19, 203, 1979.
24. Clein, L. J., *J. Neurosurg.,* 43, 337, 1975.

LATERAL AXILLARY HIATUS SYNDROME

First described by Bateman[1] in 1955, the axillary nerve can be compressed while passing through the lateral axillary hiatus in the shoulder region.

ANATOMY

The long head of the triceps muscle divides the space created by the teres major and minor, the humerus, and the scapula into two spaces: the triangular foramen or medial axillary hiatus and the quadrangular foramen or lateral axillary hiatus (Figure 1). The medial axillary hiatus lies between the teres minor muscle superiorly, the teres major muscle inferiorly, and the long head of the triceps brachii muscle laterally. Through the medial hiatus passes the circumflex scapular artery. The lateral axillary hiatus is limited proximally by the lower margin of the teres minor muscle, distally by the upper margin of the teres major muscle, laterally by the humerus, and medially by the long head of the triceps muscle. Through the lateral opening passes the axillary nerve and the posterior circumflex artery. The axillary nerve, a product of the posterior branch of the brachial plexus, enters this space from its position over the subscapular muscle; together with the posterior circumflex artery, the nerve then passes deep to the deltoid muscle. Fractures of the surgical neck of the humerus occur at this point. The axillary nerve supplies the deltoid and teres minor muscles and the skin of the posterolateral region of the shoulder and upper arm via the lateral cutaneous branch of the arm.

ETIOLOGY

Understanding the anatomy of the lateral axillary hiatus, one may foresee the potential risk of axillary nerve damage with upper arm and shoulder trauma. Fractures of the humerus and scapula as well as shoulder dislocation[2] may traumatize the neuro-vascular structures along their course. Nerve palsies may remain unnoticed until reduction of shoulder dislocations since the patient will often not move his shoulder while it is dislocated. With this as a premise, one may conclude that local tumors, organizing hematomas, or simple fracture callus may narrow the lateral axillary hiatus.

Even if sleeping, when one abducts their arm, the medial and lateral axillary hiatuses decrease in size as the teres major and minor muscles approach each other. Mansat et al.[3] postulated that this functional compression as the arm becomes perpendicular to the body may lead to nerve compression (Figure 1). Studying paraplegics with shoulder girdle hypertrophy, Kirby and Kraft[4] described simple teres hypertrophy as an etiology for nerve compression or vascular compromise. Spontaneous entrapment of the axillary nerve by fibrous band ar muscle in the quadrilateral space may occur.[5]

CLINICAL SYMPTOMS AND SIGNS

Depending on which nerve branches are compromised, the clinical signs may range from paresthesias and hypesthesias around the shoulder and upper arm to deltoid atrophy manifested by contour changes around the shoulder. Compensatory activity of the supraspinatus muscle in conjunction with the long head of the biceps helps to diminish the functional disability found with deltoid atrophy.

Electromyographical studies may indicate peripheral nerve lesions proximal to the deltoid muscle, degree of entrapment, and also reinnervation following removal of the compressive lesion. Angiography may show blockage of the posterior circumflex artery with the arm in 60° of abduction; however, this may be found in individuals without compression if the arm is abducted.

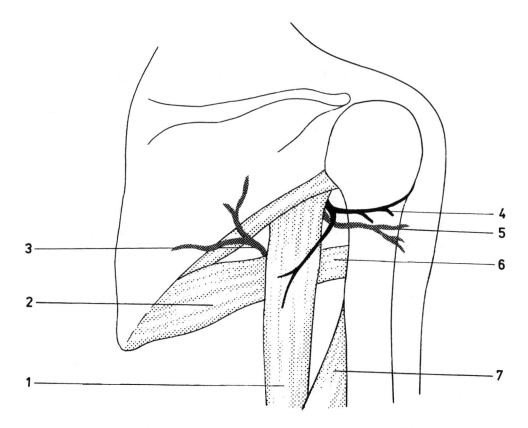

FIGURE 1.   This quadrangular space is created by the relationships of three muscle bellies and the humerus. The axillary nerve enters this space and can be damaged or compressed.

1: Long head of the triceps brachii muscle; 2: teres major muscle; 3: circumflex scapular artery; 4: axillary nerve; 5: posterior circumflex humeral artery; 6: teres major muscle; 7: medial head of the triceps brachii muscle

TREATMENT

The conservative measures of immobilization (not in abduction) and physical therapy are used prior to local injections of corticosteroids. Mumenthaler and Schliack[6] emphasize the importance of verifying reduction of the shoulder in preventing the development of this syndrome. Failure to yield improvement within 6 months indicates the need for surgical decompression. Mansat et al.[3] suggest that 40% of all patients presenting with axillary nerve compression will need surgical release of the tendinous insertions of the teres major and minor muscles. They recommend a posterior approach. If scarring has left the axillary nerve adherent to the joint, a neurolysis should be done.

REFERENCES

1. Bateman, J. E., *The Shoulder and Environs,* C. V. Mosby, St. Louis, 1955.
2. Blom, S. and Dahback, L. O., *Acta Chir. Scand.,* 136, 461, 1970.
3. Mansat, M., Mansat, Ch., and Guiraud, B., Pathologie de l'èpaule et syndromes canalaires, in *Syndromes Canalaires du Membre Supérieur,* Souquet, R., Ed., Expansion Scientifique Francaise, Paris, 1983.
4. Kirby, J. F. and Kraft, G. H., *Arch. Phys. Med. Rehabil.,* 53, 338, 1972.
5. Cahill, B. R. and Palmer, R. E., *J. Hand Surg.,* 8, 65, 1983.
6. Mumenthaler, M. and Schliack, H., *Läsionen peripherer Nerven,* G. Thieme, Stuttgart, 1965.

SUPRACONDYLAR PROCESS SYNDROME

On the anteriomedial surface of the distal humerus, an atavistic bony formation, the supracondylar process can exist and be connected to the median epicondyle by a fibrous band (Figure 1). The median nerve can be compressed in this fibro-osseus tunnel, creating the clinical symptoms of the syndrome of the supracondylar tunnel.

ANATOMY

The supracondylar process represents an anatomical variation that can be regarded as an atavistic formation found in amphibians, reptiles, and mammals.[1] This process is virtually always present in lemurs but in humans the process is only present between 0.3% and 2.7% of the time.[1,2] The bony formation starts from a large base 7 cm proximal to the medial epicondyle on the anteriomedial surface of the humerus.[3] Directed distally, its beak-like apex gives rise to a bank of connective tissue that inserts on the medial epicondyle, forming a tunnel. The process can vary from 2 to 30 mm in height.[2,4] In some lower mammals, the tunnel can be completely ossified, forming a supracondylar foramen. In humans, encrustation with calcium salts create a radiographically visible tunnel. The median nerve and brachial artery may pass through this tunnel. The ulnar nerve rarely passes under the process (Figure 2). Since the compression occurs proximal to all branches of the median nerve in the forearm, all forearm areas, both motor and sensory, innervated by the median nerve are impaired.

ETIOLOGY

Proposed etiologies for median nerve compression include the following: fractures of the supracondylar process,[1,5,6] brachial artery ischemia,[7] and idiopathic.[8,9] Domljan[10] found the median nerve to be stretched over the process like a string over a violin's bridge. Symeonides[9] described a patient who developed the syndrome after prolonged intravenous infusions with the arm fixed in extension and supination.

CLINICAL SYMPTOMS AND SIGNS

Lund[5] first described the clinical findings of this tunnel syndrome. The sensory findings consist of pain and paresthesias in the median nerve dermatomes, with deep blunt pain in the area of compression. The pain increases at night and radiates to the forearm, thumb, and first three fingers. Motor signs include weakness of the involved muscles, decreased thumb opposition, and decreased flexion of the first three fingers. In slender persons, the supracondylar process can be palpated with percussion producing a Tinel's sign, pain, and paresthesias in the median nerve's dermatomes. Thomsen[11] describes signs and symptoms in both the ulnar and median nerve distributions due to compressions in the tunnel of both nerves. Kessel and Rand[12] feel that elbow extension and forearm supination can eliminate the radial artery pulse due to compression in the tunnel.

Electromyography may be applied to diagnose impaired conduction velocity across the region.[13] Radiographic studies allow for the possibility of this diagnosis, since plan films would identify the existence of a process.

TREATMENT

Conservative therapies involved immobilization of the forearm in pronation with the elbow in $40°$ of flexion. Local corticosteroids may be helpful. Surgical decompression remains the definitive treatment, since it removes the supracondylar process.

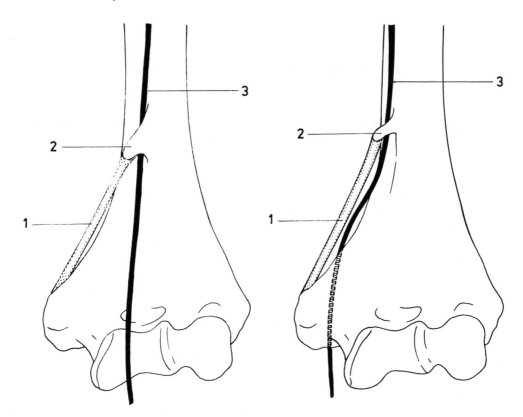

FIGURE 1.   This figure presents the location of the supracondylar process and its ligamentous attachments. 1: Connective tissue band between the supracondylar process and the medial epicondyle of the humerous; 2: supracondylar process; 3: median nerve.

FIGURE 2.   In a fashion similar to median nerve compression near the supracondylar process, the ulnar nerve may be compressed. 1: Connective tissue band; 2: supracondylar process; 3: ulnar nerve.

REFERENCES

1. Newman, A., *Am. J. Roentgenol.,* 105, 844, 1969.
2. Plavšić, B. and Cićin-Sain, S., *Lijec. Vjesn.,* 104, 231, 1982.
3. Terry, R. J., *Am. J. Phys. Antropol.,* 4, 129, 1921.
4. Zukschwerdt, L., *Fortschr. Rontgenstr.,* 40, 79, 1929.
5. Lund, H. J., *J. Bone Surg.,* 12, 925, 1930.
6. Kolb, L. V. and Moore, R. D., *J. Bone Joint Surg.,* 49 A, 532, 1967.
7. Kopell, H. P. and Thompson, W. A. L., *Peripheral Entrapment Neuropathies,* Williams and Wilkins, Baltimore, 1963.
8. Goulon, M., Lord, G., and Bedoiseau, M., *Presse Med.,* 71, 2355, 1963.
9. Symeonides, P. P., *Clin. Orthop.,* 82, 141, 1972.
10. Domljan, Z., *Lijec. Vjesn.,* 91, 959, 1969.
11. Thomsen, P. B., *Acta Orthop. Scand.,* 48, 391, 1977.
12. Kessel, L. and Rand, M., *J. Bone Joint Surg.,* 48 B, 765, 1966.
13. Smith, R. V. and Fisher, R. G., *J. Neurosurg.,* 38, 778, 1973.

PRONATOR TERES MUSCLE SYNDROME

The median nerve leaves the cubital fossa (fossa cubiti) by passing between the two heads of the pronator teres muscle and under the tendinous arch of the flexor digitorium superficialis (FDS) muscle (Figure 1). Its compression in this region produces sensory-motor symptoms of a tunnel syndrome, the syndrome of the pronator teres muscle.

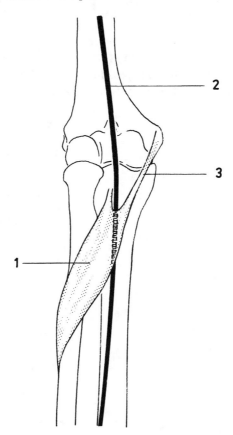

FIGURE 1.   The median nerve can run through the pronator teres muscle or between its heads during its course into the hand.
1: Pronator teres muscle; 2: median nerve; 3: humeral head of the pronator teres muscle.

ANATOMY

The median nerve passes 2.5 to 4cm below the level of the medial epicondyle between the humeral and ulnar head of the pronator teres muscle. As demonstrated by Ilić, Lolić, and Dimcević[1] and Beaton and Anson[2] the median nerve varies in its course through the pronator teres (Table 1). Upon leaving the pronator teres, the median nerve gives rise to the anterior interosseous nerve.

TABLE 1
The Findings of the Ilić, Lolić, and Dimcević (1972)[1]

Humeral and ulnar heads both present		Ulnar head missing	
Location	Percent	Location	Percent
Between the heads	56%	Behind humeral head	25%
Behind the heads	11%	Pierces muscle	3%
Through humeral head	3%		
(Per Beaton and Anson, 1939[2])	2%		
Through ulnar head	2%		

TABLE 2
Several Authors and Their Proposed Causes for the Syndrome of the Pronator Teres Muscle

Etiology	Authors
Myositis (irritating nerve)	Seyffarth, 1951[10]
Fibrous band	Fearn and Goodfellow, 1965[11] Johnson et al., 1970[3] Kopell and Thompson, 1959, 1963[12] Pesserini and Valli, 1968[13] Seyffarth, 1951[10] Sharrard, 1968[14] Thompson and Kopell, 1959[15]
Forearm trauma	Komar, 1977[16] Kopell and Thompson, 1963[12]
Dynamic relationship of the nerve and muscles in the forearm	Bora and Osterman, 1982[17] Domljan, 1969[8] Pećina, 1979[4] Thompson and Kopell, 1959[15]
Anatomical (at the aponeurosis of the FDS and biceps brachii)	Hartz et al., (1981)[5]

Having transversed the pronator teres muscle, the median nerve divides under the tendinous arch of the FDS into the layer between the FDS and the flexor digitorium profundus (FDP). It later runs between the FDS and the FDP. It then runs between the flexor carpi radialis (FCR) and the palmaris longus (PL) to reach the carpal tunnel. In the forearm, the median nerve branches multiple times to supply all wrist and hand flexors except the flexor carpi ulnaris and the ulnar portion of the FDP. Prior to entering the carpal tunnel, the median nerve gives rise to the palmaris branch, which pierces the forearm fascia to innervate the thenar eminence and the radial aspect of the wrist.

Multiple etiologies have been proposed to account for median nerve compression in the region of the pronator teres muscle (Table 2). These etiologies have a common denominator: mechanical compression secondary to static or dynamic stenosis. The presence of a fibrous band or a scarred lacertus fibrosus can create a static compression.[3]

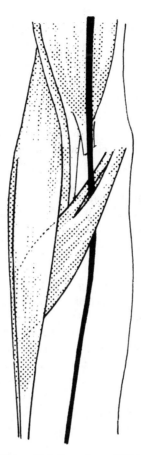

FIGURE 2.   This figure demonstrates the anatomical changes during pronator teres muscle
activity that brings its two heads together; therefore, the median nerve loses its space to run without compression.

Trauma leading to Volkmann's contracture or prolonged external compression as in
"honeymoon paralysis" have been noted to produce median nerve symptoms. Many investigators, having found static compressive agent, postulate a dynamic compression of the median
nerve during supination or elbow extension (Figure 2). In this arm position, the tendinous
portions of the muscle heads approach each other and compress the nerve.[4] In a study of 16
patients explored surgically, Hartz et al.[5] found 15 to have a compressive aponeurotic
prolongation of the biceps brachii and 13 to have a compressive tendinous arch of the
FDS.

CLINICAL SYMPTOMS AND SIGNS

Subjective symptoms and objective signs are present in the whole area of median nerve
innervation distal to the site of compression. In contrast to carpal tunnel syndrome, which
characteristically involves the muscles of the thenar eminence, the pronator teres syndrome
involves not only the thenar muscles but also the wrist and finger flexors. Patients will complain
of impaired thumb, index finger, and middle finger flexion. Sensory disturbances occur along
the volar and dorsal surfaces of the hand, the palm, and several fingers.[6]

Since the median nerve gives off the palmaris branch prior to entering the carpal tunnel,
sensory disturbances in the palm indicates compression proximal to the carpal tunnel. This is an

important diagnostic sign for differentiating between carpal tunnel syndrome and pronator teres syndrome.

CLINICAL

Spinner[7] described muscle stressing tests to localize the area of compression and entrapment. Pain and paresthesias evoked by resisted pronation of the forearm with the elbow extended implicates the heads of the pronator teres; simultaneous resisted flexion of the elbow and supination of the forearm implicates the lacertus fibrosus; and resisted flexion of the proximal interphalangeal joint of the middle finger implicates the arch of the FDS muscle belly. Pain and a Tinel's sign can also be elicited by direct pressure to the area between the two heads of the pronator teres. Therefore, patients can present after pushing cars with extended arms,[4] sudden lifting of heavy burdens,[8] or doing jobs requiring repetitive pronation and supination.

Beyond basic clinical tests, several technical tools are available. Radiographic studies may be able to identify posttraumatic lesions in the cubital region. Electromyographic examination will reveal motor unit damage and decreased conduction velocity of the FCR, FDS, and FPL.

TREATMENT

Since the majority of pronator syndromes are intermittent and mild, conservative treatment should be initially tried.[7] Treatments consist of reduction in physical activity, forearm immobilization for a limited time in neutral between supination and pronation, and local corticosteroid injection.[9] If symptoms persist, surgical decompression is required, preferably within six months of presentation. Wide exposure of the proximal forearm allows not only identification and release of the compressive structure, but also neurolysis of the median nerve if necessary. The tendinous arch between the origins of the FDS should be sectioned with release of the humeral head of the pronator teres from its radial insertion. Reviewing the results of surgical decompression in 39 patients, Hartz et al.[5] found 87% to have satisfactory results.

REFERENCES

1. Ilić, A., Lolić, V., and Dimcević, S., *Acta Orthop. Lugosl.,* 3, 193, 1971.
2. Beaton, L. E. and Anson, B. J., *Anat. Rec.,* 75, 23, 1939.
3. Johnson, R. K., Spinner, M., and Shrewsbury, M. M., *J. Hand Surg.,* 4, 48, 1970.
4. Pećina, M., *Acta Anat. (Basel),* 105, 181, 1979.
5. Hartz, C. R., Linscheid, R. L., Gramse, R. R., and Daube, J. R., *J. Bone Joint Surg.,* 63A, 885, 1981.
6. Morris, H. H. and Peters, B. H., *J. Neurol. Neurosurg. Psych.,* 39, 461, 1976.
7. Spinner, M., *Injuries to the Major Branches of Peripheral Nerves of the Forearm,* 2nd ed., Saunders, Philadelphia, 1978.
8. Domljan, Z., *Lijec. Vjesn.,* 91, 959, 1969.
9. Commandre, F., *Pathologie abarticulaire,* Lab. Cètrane, Paris, 1977.
10. Seyffarth, H., *Acta Psychiatr. Scand. Suppl.,* 74, 251, 1951.
11. Fearn, C. B. and Goodfellow, J. W., *J. Bone Joint Surg.,* 47 B, 91, 1965.
12. Kopell, H. P. and Thompson, W. A. L., *Peripheral Entrapment Neuropathies,* William Wilkinson Co., Baltimore, 1963.
13. Passerini, D. and Valli, G., *Riv. Patol. Nerv. Ment.,* 89, 1, 1968.
14. Sharrard, W. J. W., *J. Bone Joint Surg.,* 50 B, 804, 1968.
15. Thompson, W. A. L. and Kopell, H. P., *N. Engl. J. Med.,* 260, 1261, 1959.
16. Komar, J., *Alagut-szindromak,* Medicina Könyvkiado, Budapest, 1977.
17. Bora, F. W. and Osterman, A. L., *Clin. Orthop.,* 163, 20, 1982.

SUPINATOR SYNDROME
(RADIAL TUNNEL SYNDROME, SUPINATOR MUSCLE SYNDROME, AND ENTRAPMENT OF THE POSTERIOR INTEROSSEUS NERVE)

The terminal motor branch of the radial nerve may be compressed when it passes under the tendinous arch of the supinator muscle. The nerve compression and distension results in the clinical picture of the supinator syndrome described by Kopell and Thompson[1] and Mumenthaler.[2] This syndrome has also been known as posterior interosseus nerve paralysis or traumatic progressive paralysis of the deep branch of the radial nerve. Roles and Maudsley[3] describe this syndrome as radial tunnel syndrome, since they define the radial tunnel as the course of the radial nerve from its piercing of the lateral intermuscular septum, through the radial cubital sulcus, to its entrance into the supinator canal.

ANATOMY

Having perforated the lateral intermuscular septum, the radial nerve passes from posterior to anterior in the brachial sulcus and enters the sulcus cubitalis radialis, which lies between the brachialis and brachioradialis muscles. At the level of the capitellum, the radial nerve gives branches to the brachialis, brachioradialis, and extensor carpi radialis longus muscles, the periosteum of the lateral epicondyle, the humeroradial joint, and the annular ligament.[4] Within the radial cubital sulcus, the radial nerve divides into two terminal branches, the deep branch (ramus profundus) and the superficial branch (ramus superficialis).

The deep branch enters distal to the origin of the extensor carpi radialis brevis (ECRB) in the supinator canal (Figure 1). Spinner[5] noted that the margin of the ECRB may dynamically compress the deep branch during pronation before its entrance into the supinator canal. Before passing between two layers of the supinator muscle, the deep branch passes under the tendinous arch of the superficial supinator muscle layer, Frohse's arcade.[6] Frohse's arcade may exist in only 30% of adults and not at all in the fetus.[5] Entering the canal, the deep branch supplies the ECRB and the supinator muscles. The deep branch continues its lateral course around the radius to reach the dorsum of the forearm. At the distal edge of the supinator muscles, the deep branch typically divides into two divisions: (1) the muscular branch to the extensor carpi ulnaris, the extensor digitorium communis, and the extensor digiti minimis muscles; and (2) the posterior interosseus nerve to the abductor pollici longus, the extensor pollici longus, the extensor pollices brevis, and the extensor indicis muscles. The terminal branches also supply the ligaments and the capsule of the wrist.

The superficial branch of the radial nerve supplies sensory innervation to the dorsum of the hand, the first two fingers, and the radial half of the third finger.

ETIOLOGY

As listed in Table 1, multiple agents can compress the radial nerve in the supinator tunnel; however, dynamic compression due to muscular activity and anatomical relations has become one of the currently favored etiologies.[7] Compression and stretching of the nerve over Frohse's arcade occurs with repeated pronation, forearm extension, and simultaneous wrist flexion. Multiple activities have been implicated. Kopell and Thompson[1] propose that ECRB compression could lead to the supinator syndrome. Describing ten years of experience with radial tunnel syndrome, Ritts et al.[8] found the compressive agent to be the arcade of Frohse in 34 cases (57%), the ECRB in 12 cases (20%), the leash of recurrent radial vessels in 8 cases (13%), and the fibrous bands anterior to the radial head in 6 cases (10%). Sponseller and Engber[9] describe compression of the posterior interosseus nerve at both the entrance to supinator canal and the exit from the supinator muscle.

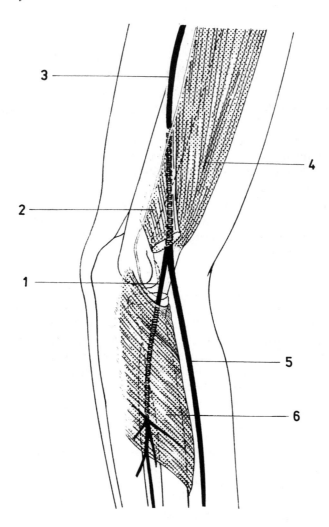

FIGURE 1.   The radial nerve runs in close proximity to multiple muscle bellies in the arm and forearm. Along its course, the nerve or its branches risk compression.
1: Deep branch (profundus) of the radial nerve; 2: brachioradialis muscle; 3: radial nerve; 4: brachialis muscle; 5: superficial branch of the radial nerve; 6: supinator muscle.

CLINICAL SYMPTOMS AND SIGNS

Deep pain in the posterior part or dorsum of the forearm followed by gradual fist weakness and local pain on compression distal to the lateral humeral epicondyle compose the clinical picture of the supinator syndrome. Unilateral and gradual in appearance, the syndrome has been described by Komar[10] as first giving rise to finger weakness, with the thumb being the last digit effected. There are no sensory deficits, since the posterior interosseus nerve has no cutaneous sensory component. The superficial branch containing the sensory fibers branches before its entrance to the supinator tunnel. Since branches to the brachioradialis and the extensor carpi radialis longus also leave before the tunnel's entrance, elbow and wrist motion remain unaffected. If the compression is stronger or longer in duration, the hand adopts the position of a hanging hand, characteristic of radial nerve paralysis.[11] Symptoms are aggravated by the simple motion of wringing the linen. While electromyographic studies can show neurological

TABLE 1
Proposed Agents and Their Respective Categories that may Compress the Radial Nerve in the Supinator Tunnel

	Cause	Author
General trauma	Radial subluxation	Grigoresco and Jordanesco, 1931[20]
	Monteggia fracture	Spinner et al., 1968[16]
	Distal humeral fracture	Esposito, 1972[21]
	Violent motion	Sharrard, 1966[15]
Tumors	Fibromas, lipomas, ganglions	Capellini, 1958[22]
		Mulholland, 1966[23]
		Richmond, 1953[24]
		Bowen and Stone, 1966[25]
		Goldman et al., 1969[11]
		Catanzariti and Cesari, 1968[26]
Inflammation	Neuroma	Whiteley and Alpers, 1959[27]
	Bursitis	Weinberger, 1939[28]
	Rheumatoid arthritis	Marmor et al., 1967[29]
		Chang et al., 1972[30]
Anatomical position	Dynamic compression	Kopell and Thomson, 1963[1]
		Spinner, 1968[5]
		Esposito, 1972[21]
	Conductor	Ritts et al., 1987[8]
	Balloonists	Guillain and Courtellemont, 1905[31]
	Violinists	Silverstein, 1937[32]
	Wimmers	Kruse, 1958[33]

compromise, Zeuke et al.[12] believe that surgical treatment can be based on the characteristic clinical picture alone.

In spite of a characteristic picture, the supinator tunnel syndrome is often not recognized or is mistaken for radial epicondylitis — tennis elbow.[13] These two syndromes may appear together, and Moss and Switzer[14] have described a variety of symptoms associated with resistant tennis elbow and resistent radial tunnel pain. The same motions of pronation, forearm extension, and wrist flexion common to the supinator syndrome also occurs at the end of the serve in tennis, thus the term tennis elbow. Pain over the lateral epicondyle with resisted middle finger extension with an extended arm can be confused with the local tenderness distal to the lateral epicondyle found in a patient with supinator syndrome.

TREATMENT

Treatment seeks to avoid repetitive trauma to the nerve in the tunnel. Physical therapy and local corticosteroid injections give good results if dynamic compression is not a factor. Surgical treatment should not be postponed too long, since irreversible nerve damage may occur.[5,15-17] Palazzi et al.[18] recommend surgical intervention within the first four months of symptoms. Since the clinical picture of radial epicondylitis and supinator syndrome can overlap, Roles and Maudsley[3] recommend decompression of the deep branch of the radial nerve in the supinator tunnel when treating resistant epicondylitis. Believing that 30% of patients with radial epicondylitis have posterior interosseus compression, Jalovaara and Lindholm's[19] primary surgical approach is decompression of the posterior interosseous nerve when presented with resistant radial epicondylitis.

REFERENCES

1. Kopell, H. P. and Thompson, W. A. L., *Peripheral Entrapment Neuropathies,* Williams and Wilkins, Baltimore, 1963.
2. Mumenthaler, M. and Schliack, H., *Läsionen peripherer Nerven,* Georg Thieme, Stuttgart, 1965.
3. Roles, N. C. and Maudsley, R. H., *J. Bone Joint Surg.,* 54B, 499, 1972.
4. Kaplan, E. B., *J. Bone Joint Surg.,* 41A, 147, 1959.
5. Spinner, M., *J. Bone Joint Surg.,* 50B, 809, 1968.
6. Fröhse, F. and Fränkel, M., *Die Muskeln des menschlichen Armes,* G. Fischer, Jena, 1908.
7. Capener, N., *J. Bone Joint Surg.,* 48B, 770, 1966.
8. Ritts, D. G., Wood, B. M., and Linscheid, L. R., *Clin. Orthop.,* 219, 201, 1987.
9. Sponseller, P.D. and Engber, D. W., *J. Hand Surg.,* 8, 420, 1983.
10. Komar, J., *Alagut-szindromak,* Medicina Könyvkiado, Budapest, 1977.
11. Goldman, S., Hornet, J. C., Sobel, R., and Goldstein, A. S., *Arch. Neurol.,* 21, 435, 1969.
12. Zeuke, W., Arnold, H., and Heidrich, R., *Schweiz. Arch. Neurol. Neurochir. Psychiat.,* 113, 99, 1973.
13. Domljan, Z., *Lijec. Vjesn.,* 91, 959, 1969.
14. Moss, H. S. and Switzer, E. H., *J. Hand Surg.,* 8, 414, 1983.
15. Sharrard, W. J. W., *J. Bone Joint Surg.,* 48B, 777, 1966.
16. Spinner, M., Freundlich, B. D., and Teicher, J., *Clin. Orthop.,* 58, 141, 1968.
17. Durandeau, A. and Geneste, R., *Rev. Chir. Orthop.* (Suppl. II), 74, 156, 1988.
18. Palazzi, S., Palazzi, C., Raimondi, P., and Araburo, F., Syndromes compressifs du nerf radial, in *Syndromes Canalaires du Membre Supérieur,* Souquet, R., Ed., Expansion Scientifique Francaise, Paris, 1983.
19. Jalovaara, P. and Lindholm, R. V., *Arch. Orthop. Trauma Surg.,* 108, 243, 1989.
20. Grigoresco, D. and Jordanesco, C., *Rev. Neurol.,* 2, 102, 1931.
21. Esposito, G. M., *N.Y. St. J. Med.,* 72, 717, 1972.
22. Capellini, O., *Chir. Organi Mov.,* 45, 338, 1958.
23. Mulholland, R. C., *J. Bone Joint Surg.,* 48B, 781, 1966.
24. Richmond, D. A., *J. Bone Joint Surg.,* 35B, 83, 1953.
25. Bowen, T. L. and Stone, K. H., *J. Bone Joint Surg.,* 48B, 774, 1966.
26. Catanzariti, G. and Cesari, F., *Clin. Orthop.,* 20, 512, 1968.
27. Whiteley, W. H. and Alpers, B. J., *Arch. Neurol.,* 1, 226, 1959.
28. Weinberger, L. M., *Surg. Gynecol. Obstet.,* 69, 358, 1939.
29. Marmor, L., Lawrence, J. F., and Dubois, E. L., *J. Bone Joint Surg.,* 49A, 381, 1967.
30. Chang, L. W., Gowans, J. D. C., Granger, C. V., and Milender, L. H., *Arthritis Rheum.,* 15, 350, 1972.
31. Guillain, G. and Courtellemont, H., *Presse Méd.,* 13, 50, 1905.
32. Silverstein, A., *Arch. Neurol. Psychiatry,* 38, 885, 1937.
33. Kruse, F., *Neurology,* 8, 307, 1958.

ANTERIOR INTEROSSEOUS SYNDROME
(KILOH-NEVIN SYNDROME)

A motor branch of the median nerve in the cubital region, the anterior interosseous nerve risks compression throughout its course in the forearm (Figure 1). Kiloh and Nevin[1] first described two patients with classical prevention of the decreased function of the distal phalanx of both the thumb and the index finger.

ANATOMY

From the posterior surface of the median nerve 2 to 8 cm distal to the medial humeral epicondyle originates an exclusively motor nerve branch, the anterior interosseous (palmaris) nerve. While initially paralleling the median nerve, the anterior interosseous nerve soon dives under the deep fascial layer of the flexor digitorum superficialis (FDS) to run along the interosseous membrane between the flexor policies longus (FPL) laterally and flexor digitorum profundus (FDP) medially. It is accompanied by interosseal vessels. Distally the nerve ends under the pronator quadratus (PQ), branching 2 to 5 cm distal to its origin. The anterior interosseous nerve supplies the FPL, the FDP to the second finger, and the PQ.[2] Some authors mention the possibility of direct innervation by the median or ulnar nerve. As a separate entity or a component, the anterior interosseous nerve may accompany the median nerve and course between the heads of the pronator teres or between the tendinous arch of the FDS. Because of these anatomical relationships, some authors[3,4] do not differentiate the pronator teres syndrome from the anterior interosseous syndrome. However, the Kiloh-Nevin syndrome defines only anterior interosseous nerve involvement and, thus, is only a motor deficiency.

ETIOLOGY

The description of the anterior interosseous syndrome as a tunnel syndrome remains a question of definition. In which tunnel does the nerve run? Several authors have reported varied etiologies for nerve compression (Table 1).

These etiologies can range from median nerve tumors causing isolated paralysis to fibrous anomalies of the FPL and FDS. Englert[5] and Haussmann[6] have described this syndrome as arising without any external compression. Operatively, the fibers of the anterior interosseous nerve have been found to be compressed within the main trunk of the median nerve proximal to the elbow. These two cases of intratruncal fascicular compression were treated in one case by neurolysis and in the other case by translocation.

Penkert[7] mentions the possibility that trauma along the nerve's course may lead to segmental demyelination and paresis. Paresis disappears gradually with remyelinization. While the anterior interosseous nerve may be compressed as it pierces the fascia of the FDS, most authors reject this hypothesis, since this fascial is a loose structure. Since the nerve passes under the radial portion of the tendinous arch of the FDS, Luppino et al.[2] and Penkert[7] describe the upper margin of this arch as the compressive agent of the tunnel. Nerve recovery after arch sectioning confirms this hypothesis. However, as Eren et al.[8] described, only half of the 40 surgical patients reported in the literature had identifiable compressive causes.[6-16]

CLINICAL SYMPTOMS AND SIGNS

While developing acutely or gradually, the clinical picture is manifested by an inability of the patient to pinch between his thumb and index finger. This characteristic pinch sign (Figure 2) develops from impaired flexion of the terminal phalanges of the thumb and of the index finger. Thus, the patient pinches with extended distal interphalangeal joints. Opposition of the thumb

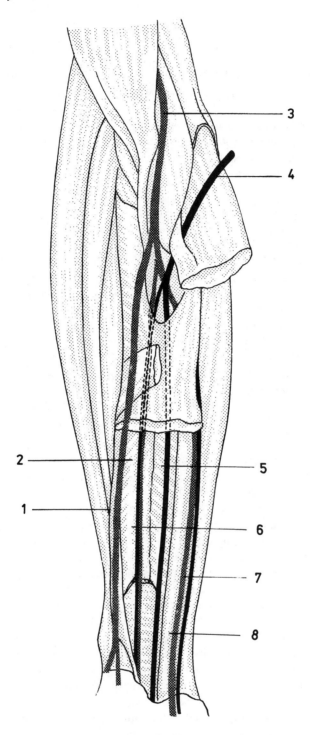

FIGURE 1.   The forearm contains multiple muscle groups that are
intertwined with the entire neurovascular supply to the hand. The
close proximity of all of these structures dictates that variations in the
normal structure of one will affect the other associated structures.
1: Radial artery; 2: anterior interosseus nerve; 3: brachial artery; 4:
median nerve; 5: median nerve; 6: anterior interosseus nerve; 7: ulnar
nerve; 8: ulnar artery.

TABLE 1
Various Etiologies for Nerve Compression

Etiology	Author
Trauma/forearm fractures	Warren, 1963[24]
	Luppino et al., 1972[2]
	Penkert, 1983[7]
Post-traumatic thrombosis of the antibrachial vessels	Haussmann, 1982[6]
Vascular anomalies	Eren et al., 1983[8]
Neuroma of the median nerve	Spinner, 1970[22]
Anatomical anomalies	Spinner, 1970[22]
	Benini and Tedesci, 1974[25]
	Gardner-Thorpe, 1974[26]
	Leven and Hauffman, 1976[27]
Intratruncal fascicular compression	Englert, 1976[5]
	Haussmann, 1982[6]
Segmental demyelination	Penkert, 1983[7]

and finger flexion of the 3rd, 4th, and 5th digits remain intact. However, the ability to write is usually lost.[17] Additionally, the patient cannot clench his fist (Figure 3). The syndrome may be complete with both the thumb and finger affected, or incomplete with either the thumb or finger affected. Hill et al.[18] have reported the largest series of incomplete syndromes with a total of 26 patients from both the U.S. and Canada. Occasionally, the patient will have weakness of the pronator quadratus muscle (PQ). The PQ must be examined with the elbow flexed to eliminate the effect of the pronator teres.[19] Patients feel dull pain into the proximal third of the forearm that is aggravated by radial pressure at the level of the tendinous arch of the FDS. Characteristically, there is no sensory loss nor sign. The presence of sensory symptoms should indicate median nerve compromise.

Electromyography will show not only denervation of the affected muscles, but also reinnervation if it occurs. Eren et al.[8] have found a tendency for spontaneous recovery within six months.

TREATMENT

As in most tunnel syndromes, conservative therapy may be applied early in the disease course, with a maximum time limit in which to see if relief is achieved. This limit is typically six months after the onset of symptoms if there is no evidence of recovery, either clinically or electrodiagnostically. Eren et al.[8] found that five of seven patients in their series recovered spontaneously. Therefore, in the absence of a definitive cause of compression, conservative therapy may allow time for reinnervation.

Assmus et al.[20] proceeds to surgical decompression if there is no evidence of recovery within two months. Other surgeons extend their follow-up to three to six months with electromyographic evaluation [21,22] Surgical treatment may include exploration with fibrous band or tendon release, removal of anomalous muscles, or neurolysis.[22,23]

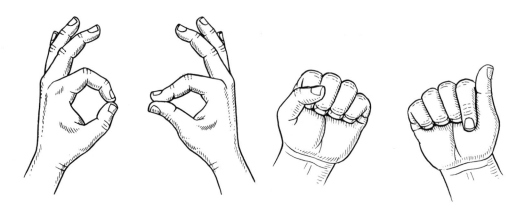

FIGURE 2.   This figure compares the pinch of the unaffected hand with the pinch of a hand where the anterior
interosseus nerve is compromised (pinch sign).

FIGURE 3.   Inability to complete one's fist due to problems incorporating the thumb and index finger may give
the investigator a solid clinical sign for nerve compression.

REFERENCES

1. Kiloh, L.G. and Nevin, S., *Br. Med. J.,* 1, 850, 1952.
2. Luppino, T., Celli, L., and Monteleone, M., *Chir. Organi Mov.,* 61, 89, 1972.
3. Komar, J., *Alagut-szindromak,* Medicina Könyvkiado, Budapest, 1977.
4. Commandre, F., *Pathologie Abarticulaire,* Lab. Cëtrane, Paris, 1977.
5. Englert, H. M., *Handchirurgie,* 8, 61, 1976.
6. Haussmann, P., *Handchirurgie,* 14, 183, 1982.
7. Penkert, G., *Handchirurgie,* 15, 223, 1983.
8. Eren, S., Brùser, P., and Meyer-Clement, M., *Handchirurgie,* 15, 221, 1983.
9. Havelius, L. and Tuverson, T., *Arch. Orthop. Traumat. Surg.,* 96, 59, 1980.
10. Nigst, H. and Dick, W., *Arch. Orthop. Traumat. Surg.,* 93,307, 1979.
11. Omer, G. E., *J. Bone Joint Surg.,* 56A, 1615, 1974.
12. Penkert, G. and Schwandt, *Handchirurgie,* 72, 79, 1980.
13. Rask, M. R., *Clin. Orthop.,* 142, 176, 1979.
14. Stern, M. B., Rosner, L. J., and Blinderman, E. E., *Clin. Orthop.,* 53, 95, 1967.
15. Thomas, D. F., *J. Bone Joint Surg.,* 44B, 962, 1962.
16. Vichare, N. A., *J. Bone Joint Surg.,* 50B, 806, 1968.
17. Stern, M. B., *Clin. Orthop.,* 187, 223, 1984.
18. Hill, N. J., Howard, F. M., and Huffer, B. R., *J. Hand Surg. [AM.],* 10, 4, 1985.
19. Bora, F. W. and Osterman, A. L., *Clin. Orthop.,* 163, 20B, 1982.
20. Assmus, H. J., Hamer, J., and Martin, K., *Nervenarzt,* 46, 659, 1975.
21. Nakano, K. K. and Lundergan, C., et al., *Arch. Neurol.,* 34, 477, 1977.
22. Spinner, M., *J. Bone Joint Surg.,* 52A, 84, 1970.
23. Werner, C. O., *Int. Orthop.,* 13, 193, 1989.
24. Warren, J. D., *J. Bone Joint Surg.,* 45B, 511, 1963.
25. Benini, A. and Tedeschi, N., *Schweiz. Med. Wochenschr.,* 104, 1695, 1974.
26. Gardner-Thorpe, Ch., *J. Neurol. Neurosurg. Psych.,* 37, 1146, 1974.
27. Leven, B. and Hauffmann, G., *Nervenarzt,* 47, 502, 1976.

SULCUS ULNARIS SYNDROME

During its course down the arm, the ulnar nerve lies in a sulcus on the posterior surface of the medial humeral epicondyle. Compression of the ulnar nerve in this area presents with symptoms characteristic of the syndrome of the ulnar nerve sulcus.

ANATOMY

As shown in Figure 1, the ligament connecting the medial epicondyle to the olecranon covers the ulnar nerve, creating a fibro-osseus tunnel. This ligament serves to prevent subluxation of the ulnar nerve with forearm motion. Distal to the tunnel, the ulnar nerve branches to supply the motor innervation to the following muscles: flexor carpi ulnaris, the ulnar component of the flexor digitorum profundus, the hypothenar muscles, the interossei muscles, the two most ulnar lumbricals, the adductor pollicis, and the deep head of the flexor pollicis brevis. Sensory branches to the fingers and hand originate distal to the sulcus.

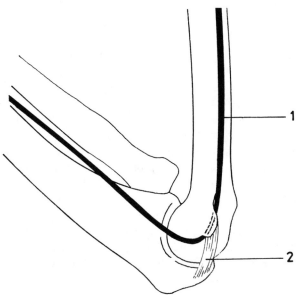

FIGURE 1.   The ulnar nerve may be compressed proximal to the elbow near the medial epicondyle. A ligament connecting the medial epicondyle with the olecranon can be suspect.
1: Ulnar nerve; 2: epicondylo-olecranon ligament.

ETIOLOGY

Trauma, the consequences of trauma, and rheumatic changes in the region of the medial epicondyle can compress the ulnar nerve by narrowing the fibro-osseus tunnel. Vidal et al.[1] describes two peaks: a peak between ages 20 and 30 years with trauma as the predominating cause, and a second peak between ages 50 and 60 years with rheumatic and degenerative joint disease predominating.

As an etiology, trauma can range from posttraumatic cubitus valgus to chronic nerve compression. Cubitus valgus can cause paresthesias and other sensory disturbances without affecting the cubital joint. Patients who lean on their elbows at work or while confined to bed may develop ulnar nerve compression at the elbow. The basic damage remains nerve damage either due to compression or direct contusions. Microtrauma or repetitive nerve stretches sustained in such varied activities as baseball, construction (jack hammers), boxing, or javelin throwing[2] may traumatize the ulnar nerve. Supracondylar fractures, distal humeral fractures, elbow dislocations, callus formation, and surgical exploration of these areas all may lead to direct or indirect trauma to the nerve in its tunnel. Rheumatic diseases lead to joint degeneration and distort the normal anatomy of the elbow. Thus, the ulnar nerve finds itself stretched or compressed along its course.

While not a true tunnel syndrome, subluxation of the ulnar nerve may present with similar symptoms, since it results in nerve compression; however, compression occurs secondary to an enlarged tunnel rather than a compressed one.[3] Described by many authors,[4-7] ulnar nerve subluxation occurs as the elbow flexes and the nerve glides medially to be tensioned against the medial epicondyle. Mumenthaler and Schliack[5] described subluxation secondary to traumatic edema of the nerve, which forced the nerve to leave the tunnel.

The table below lists the hypotheses of several investigators as to the etiologies of ulnar nerve subluxation.

Cause	Author(s)
Rupture of the epicondylo-olecranon ligament	Platt, 1926;[8] Arkin, 1940;[9] Godshall and Hansen, 1971[10]
Cubitus valgus	Marinescu and Danalia, 1968[11]
Shallow sulcus	Rolfsen, 1970[3]
Congenital anomalies of the medial epicondyle	Wachsmuth and Wilhelm, 1968[12]

CLINICAL SYMPTOMS AND SIGNS

In the first stage of the syndrome, paresthesias, hyperesthesia, hypesthesia, and pain develop in the sensory dermatome of the ulnar nerve. Paresthesias and pain may also be found proximally near the shoulder as the compression progresses. Tinel's sign, produced by tapping over the ulnar sulcus, may not be positive. Hypotrophy and atrophy may be found if the nerve compression remains unrelieved. Muscle wasting may be first seen in the web space between the first and second metacarpals followed by interossei and hypothenar wasting. Loss of ulnar innervation will lead to a claw-hand appearance.

Radiographic studies may allow visualization of rheumatic, arthritic, or post-traumatic changes around the elbow. Serology and laboratory testing may distinguish between several rheumatologic etiologies if present. Electromyography and conduction velocity determination will contribute to isolating the location of the compression.

TREATMENT

Conservative therapy remains similar to that of many other tunnel syndromes: rest, removal of the causative agent, and local corticosteroid injection. The sulcus may be injected in the center of an imaginary line connecting the medial epicondyle to the medial edge of the olecranon. Surgical treatment consists of releasing the ligament connecting the epicondyle and the olecranon, ligament release and medial epicondylectomy, or anterior transposition of the ulnar nerve.[13] First performed successfully in 1898 by Curtis,[14] transposition has been successfully adopted by many surgeons,[1,15] including the editors. Studying clinical and electromyographical results following various surgical decompressions of the ulnar nerve, Deutinger et al.[16] found that anterior transposition of the ulnar nerve yielded the best results. One must note that surgical decompression must occur before permanent nerve damage results; otherwise, the type of surgical release performed will not change the outcome.

REFERENCES

1. Vidal, J., Allieu, Y., Connes, H., and Horwath, T., *Ann. Orthoped. L'Ouest,* 6, 27, 1974.
2. Del Pizzo, W., Jobe, W. F., and Norwood, L., *Am. J. Sports* Med., 5, 182, 1977.
3. Komar, J., *Alagut-szindromak,* Medicina Könyvkiado, Budapest, 1977.
4. Childress, H. M., *J. Bone Joint Surg.,* 38A, 978, 1956.
5. Mumenthaler, M. and Schliack, H., *Läsionen peripherer Nerven,* G. Thieme, Stuttgart, 1965.
6. Domljan, Z., *Lijec. Vjesn.,* 91, 959, 1969.
7. Commandre, F., *Pathologie Abarticulaire,* Laboratoire Cérane, Paris, 1977.
8. Platt, H., *Br. J. Surg.,* 13, 409, 1926.
9. Arkin, A. M., *J. Mt. Sinai Hosp.,* 7, 208, 1940.
10. Godshall, R. W. and Hansen, C. A., *J. Bone Joint Surg.,* 53A, 359, 1971.
11. Marinescu, V. and Danaila, L., *Neurol. Psychiatr. Neurochir.,* 13, 229, 1968.
12. Wachsmuth, W. and Wilhelm, A., *Monatsschr. Unfallheilkd.,* 71, 1, 1968.
13. Froimson, A. and Zahrawi, F., *J. Hand Surg.,* 5, 391, 1980.
14. Curtis, B. F., *J. Nerv. Ment. Dis.,* 25, 480, 1898.
15. Bora, F. W. and Osterman, A. L., *Clin. Orthop.,* 163, 20, 1982.
16. Deutinger, M., Mayr, N., Frey, N., Mandl, H., Holle, J., and Freilinger, G., *Z. Orthop.,* 127, 639, 1989.

FLEXOR CARPI ULNARIS MUSCLE SYNDROME
(CUBITAL TUNNEL SYNDROME)

Commonly known by some as the cubital tunnel syndrome, the syndrome of the flexor carpi ulnaris muscle includes ulnar nerve compression, since it courses not only in its sulcus behind the medial humeral epicondyle but also between the two heads of the flexor carpi ulnaris muscle. Feindel and Stratford[1] described ulnar nerve compression in the latter situation as the cubital tunnel syndrome. However to avoid confusion, this book will use the more inclusive definition to avoid confusion and accurately define the region in question.

ANATOMY

The ulnar nerve leaves the ulnar sulcus behind the medial humeral epicondyle and passes between the humeral and ulnar heads of the flexor carpi ulnaris (Figure 1). A tendinous arch, the arcuate ligament, connects these heads and defines the tunnel's entrance and roof. Extending from the medial epicondyle to the medial border of the olecranon, the triangularly shaped arcuate ligament additionally serves as a common origin for both the humeral and the ulnar heads of the flexor carpi ulnaris muscle.

Once in the forearm, the ulnar nerve lies between the flexor digitorum superficialis, the flexor digitorum profundus, and the flexor carpi ulnaris muscles. The ulnar vessels join the ulnar nerve in this region by transversing the cubital tunnel, which is defined as lying under the tendinous arch connecting the radial and humeral heads of the flexor digitorum superficialis muscle. Use of the term cubital tunnel syndrome in regard to the ulnar nerve could lead to more confusion in this setting.

Sensory and motor branches leaving the canal at the level of the origin of the flexor carpi ulnaris muscle are identical to those branches originating in the ulnar sulcus behind the medial epicondyle. Therefore, the differential diagnosis between compression in the ulnar sulcus and the flexor carpi ulnaris becomes more difficult.

ETIOLOGY

The anatomical relationships around the elbow affecting the ulnar nerve both in the ulnar sulcus and between the two heads of the flexor carpi ulnaris muscle are similar; therefore, several of the etiologies are similar. However, an idiopathic form of the syndrome of the flexor carpi ulnaris relies on the anatomical relationship of its heads and its tendinous arch. First described by Feindel and Stratford,[1] the fibrous arch compresses the nerve as elbow flexion tenses the arch. Several other investigators have described the arch's importance.[2-4] Consistent with Esposito's[5] finding of a 10% tunnel volume reduction in flexion, cadaver studies have demonstrated an increase in compartment pressures from 7 to 24 mm Hg when the elbow changes from extension to flexion.[6] Using this finding, Buehler and Thayer[7] have endorsed the "elbow flexion test" as a clinical test for nerve compression. Vanderpool et al.[8] described a change in the anatomical head relationship when the elbow flexes. Extrapolating from this finding one can understand how this syndrome may appear more frequently in those who work for many hours with their elbows flexed as described by Kenneth.[9] Another cadaver study by Amadio and Beckenbaugh[10] found that the deep aponeurosis of the flexor carpi ulnaris muscle was a potential site for nerve compression.

While functional anatomical changes may account for many of the patients with this syndrome, other etiologies have been postulated. Thompson and Kopell[11] emphasize the importance of external trauma, since the nerve lies quite superficially. Arthritis of the elbow may produce a compressive proliferative synovitis and bony osteophytes. Loose bodies and other

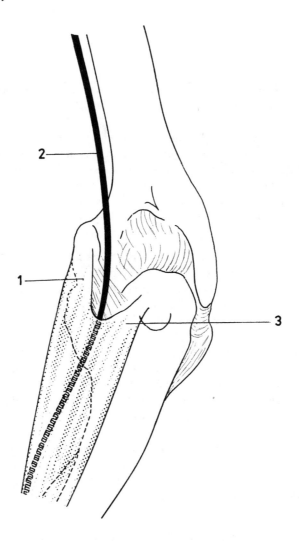

FIGURE 1.   The ulnar nerve may also be compressed just distal
to the elbow by the heads of the flexor carpi ulnaris muscle.
1: Humeral head of the flexor carpi ulnaris muscle; 2: ulnar nerve;
3: ulnar head of the flexor carpi ulnaris muscle.

synovial changes have also been submitted as causes. Tumors, ganglions, perineural cysts, and
lipomas, in addition to anomalous muscles and variations in the anconeus muscle may be rare
causes of nerve compression.[13] Vidal et al.[14] described three cases that did not fit any aforementioned etiology.

CLINICAL SYMPTOMS AND SIGNS

Gradual development of paresthesias, pain, and muscle weakness have led to description
of this syndrome as tardy ulnar nerve palsy. In the end stage, paresis of ulnar innervated
musculature leads to the development of the Froment's sign (Figure 2). This sign requires
dysfunction of the adductor pollicis muscle. While having the patient hold a piece of paper
between the thumb and index finger, the physician will observe compensation by the flexor
pollicis longus muscle. Thus, the interphalangeal joint of the thumb will be held in flexion. While
this finding is diagnostic of ulnar nerve damage, atrophy and this sign occur more frequently

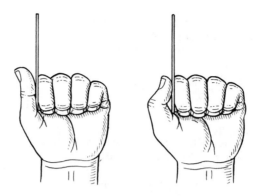

FIGURE 2.   Froment's sign.

in the syndrome of the flexor carpi ulnaris muscle than in any other ulnar nerve compressive syndrome.[15] A Tinel's sign will be appreciated more distally in this syndrome than in the syndrome of the ulnar sulcus. Radiographic studies and a thorough history may indicate when prior fractures in development have led to an elbow deformity that alters the nerve's course.[16] Electromyographic studies will usually indicate a pathology near the elbow. Szendroi et al.[17] postulate that Dupuytren's contracture is a late consequence of this syndrome.

Neurologic symptoms and signs similar to ulnar nerve entrapment can be caused by brachial plexus compression from thoracic outlet syndrome or an occult apical lung tumor. However, neither a Tinel's sign nor a localized electromyographical change will be appreciated at the elbow.[18] Epicondylitis may be mistaken for this syndrome.[19] However, epicondylitis (or epitrochleitis, since the medial epicondyle lies above the humeral trochlea) presents as a localized pain on palpation without paresis or sensory changes in the ulnar nerve distribution.

TREATMENT

Advised for patients with intermittent mild symptoms without neurological deficits,[20] conservative therapies include short-term immobilization, physical therapy, and local corticosteroid infiltration. In the presence of conservative therapy failure or more definite neurological signs of compromise, one must proceed immediately with surgical release. Except with respect to sectioning of the tendinous arch of the flexor carpi ulnaris muscle, no absolute consensus exists with respect to what release to perform; therefore the releases performed are as follows: anterior subcutaneous or submuscular transposition of the ulnar nerve,[21-23] medial epicondylectomy,[24] and simple tunnel decompression if this is the only site of entrapment.[25,26] Release of the flexor's tendinous arch usually disturbs the ligament connecting the olecranon and epicondyle. Since compression in the ulnar sulcus may masquerade as flexor carpi ulnaris muscle compression, both decompression in both locations and anterior translocation of the ulnar nerve are recommended. If ulnar nerve decompression is not verified, many patients will present repeatedly, greatly increasing their risks of complication. Higher success rates have been found with translocation and decompression when compared to simple decompression.[23,24,27] Surgical intervention must be planned according to the specific indications of each patient,[28-31] since no single surgical intervention may be ideal. Complications of surgical intervention include the following: neuroma of the medial antebrachial cutaneous nerve; subluxation or dislocation of the nerve after release or transposition; inadequate protective covering for the nerve after transposition; unrecognized residual tethers, which may lead to new sites for compression; iatrogenic nerve injury; incomplete decompression; and compression secondary to postoperative scar formation.[8,32]

REFERENCES

1. Feindel, W. and Stratford, J., *Can. Med. Assoc. J.,* 78, 51, 1958.
2. Ho, K. C. and Marmor, L., *Am. J. Surg.,* 121, 355, 1971.
3. Howard, M. F., *Orthop. Clin. North Am.,* 17, 375, 1986.
4. Nicolle, F. V. and Noolhouse, F. M., *J. Trauma,* 5, 313, 1965.
5. Esposito, G. M., *N.Y. St. J. Med.,* 72717, 1972.
6. Pechan, J. and Julis, I., *J. Biomech.,* 8, 75, 1975.
7. Buehler, M. J. and Thayer, T. D., *Clin. Orthop.,* 233, 213, 1988.
8. Vanderpool, D. W., Chalmers, J., Lamb, D. W., and Whiston, T. B., *J. Bone Joint Surg.,* 50B, 792, 1968.
9. Kenneth, W. E. P., *Can. J. Surg.,* 13, 255, 1970.
10. Amadio, P. C. and Beckenbaugh, R. D., *J. Hand Surg.,* 11, 83, 1986.
11. Thompson, W. A. L. and Kopell, H. P., *N. Engl. J. Med.,* 260, 1261, 1959.
12. Macicol, M. F., *Hand,* 1, 14, 1982.
13. Spinner, M., *Injuries to the Major Branches of Peripheral Nerves of the Forearm,* 2nd ed., Saunders, Philadelphia, 1978.
14. Vidal, J., Allieu, Y., Connes, H., and Horworth, T., *Ann. Orthopéd. l'Ouest,* 6, 27, 1974.
15. Eisen, A., *Neurology,* 24, 256, 1974.
16. Holmes, J. C. and Hall, J. E., *Clin. Orthop.,* 135, 128, 1978.
17. Szendroi, M., Hasznos, T., and Galambos, J., *Handchirurgie,* 3, 3, 1971.
18. Hirsh, F. L. and Thanki, A., *Postgrad. Med.,* 77, 211, 1985.
19. Bora, F. W. and Osterman, A.L., *Clin. Orthop.,* 153, 20, 1982.
20. Dawson, D. M., Hallett, M., and Millender, L. H., *Entrapment Neuropathies,* Little and Brown, Boston, Toronto, 1983.
21. Inserra, S. and Spinner, M., *J. Hand Surg.,* 11, 80, 1986.
22. Learsmonth, J. R., *Surg. Gynecol. Obstet.,* 75, 792, 1942.
23. Leffert, R. D., *J. Hand Surg.,* 7, 147, 1982.
24. Craven, P. R. and Green, D. P., *J. Bone Joint Surg.,* 62A, 986, 1980.
25. Osborne, G. V., *J. Bone Joint Surg.,* 39B, 782, 1957.
26. Wilson, D. H. and Krout, R., *J. Neurosurg.,* 38, 780, 1973.
27. McGowan, A. J., *J. Bone Joint Surg.,* 32B, 293, 1950.
28. Taylor, J. K., personal communications.
29. Lugnegard, H., Walheim, G., and Wennbert, A., *Acta Orthop. Scand.,* 48, 168, 1977.
30. MacNicol, M. F., *J. Bone Joint Surg.,* 61B, 159, 1979.
31. Foster, R. J. and Edshage, S., *J. Hand Surg.,* 6, 181, 1981.
32. Nigst, H., *Handchirurgie,* 15, 212, 1983.

SYNDROME OF THE MUSCULOCUTANEOUS NERVE
AT THE ELBOW

Compression of the musculocutaneous nerve near the elbow has been recently described by Bassett and Nunley[1] based on 11 patients. Sensory disturbances occur when the nerve is compressed as it pierces the brachial fascia.

ANATOMY

Originating from the lateral cord of the brachial plexus, the musculocutaneous nerve supplies motor branches to the coracobrachialis, biceps brachii, and brachialis muscles and sensory branches to portions of the forearm and wrist. The lateral cord of the brachial plexus crosses into the axilla before dividing into the musculocutaneous and a contribution to the median nerve. The musculocutaneous nerve stays lateral to the axillary artery, and lies on the coracobrachialis before piercing through the muscle. In 10% of the cases, the nerve does not pierce the muscle's fascia. The nerve, then, continues to run between the biceps brachii and brachioradialis muscles before piercing the brachial fascia 2 to 5 cm proximal to the medial cubital crease. Olson[2] described the nerve as continuing its course under the lateral margin of the biceps tendon until the cubital crease. Shown in Figure 1, the musculocutaneous nerve becomes the lateral antebrachial cutaneous nerve, which courses distally under the cephalic vein. While terminology may vary, the lateral antebrachial cutaneous nerve splits to form the palmar and the dorsal branches. The palmar branch supplies the anterior skin of the lateral (radial) half of the forearm before terminating at the thenar eminence. The dorsal or posterior branch runs along the radial margin of the forearm to supply the posterior surface of the distal third of the forearm before terminating at the base of the first metacarpal bone.

ETIOLOGY

Compression of the lateral antebrachial cutaneous nerve may occur when the nerve passes below the tendon of the biceps muscle before piercing the brachial fascia. According to Bassett and Nunley,[1] the lateral free margin of the biceps aponeurosis compresses the nerve against the brachial fascia with elbow extension. Pronation further increases nerve compression. Eight of eleven patients developed symptoms in the dominant hand.[1] All 11 had histories of acute or chronic trauma to the elbow usually consisting of forced elbow extension coupled with forearm pronation. Other cases have been reported with tennis backhand strokes,[3] repeated pronation and supination of the forearm, and excessive screw driving during house construction (3000 screws by hand). Braddom and Wolfe[4] have reported acute entrapment of the musculocutaneous nerve proximally under the edge of a hypertrophied coracobrachialis muscle. However, in addition to sensory losses, the patient had paresis of the biceps, brachialis, and coracobrachialis muscles following very strenuous physical exercise.

CLINICAL SYMPTOMS AND SIGNS

The diagnosis of the syndrome of the musculataneous nerve in the region of the elbow can be confused with the symptoms of epicondylitis, especially since both syndromes can be linked to tennis. Pain is always present and usually located in the anterolateral portion of the elbow. In the patients who develop acute compression, their pain is usually burning in nature. Patients avoid full elbow extension with forearm pronation, since this motion aggravates their pain. Supination may offer some relief from pain. Patients with chronic trauma present with varying pain and hypesthesia in the wrist and the forearm. Patients do not usually recognize the extent of their hypesthesia; however, they are tender over the musculocutaneous nerve in the region

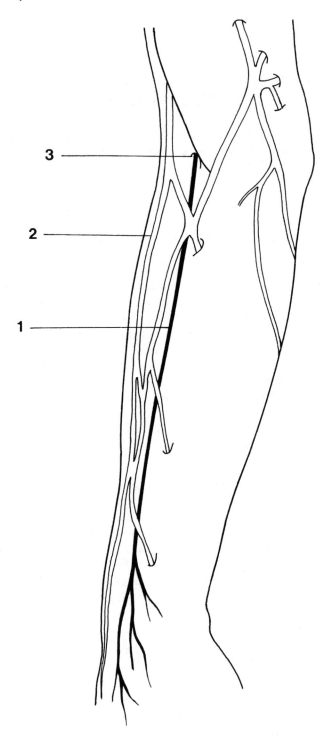

FIGURE 1.   Because it runs superficially, the terminal portion of the musculocutaneous nerve may be damaged.
1: Lateral cutaneous nerve of the forearm; 2: cephalic vein; 3: origin of the musculocutaneous nerve as it exits through a layer of fascia underlying the skin.

under the biceps muscle where it pierces the brachial fascia. In the subacute and chronic forms, patients have pain with forearm pronation with an extended elbow.

TREATMENT

Treatment options include the following: rest; avoidance of motions provoking pain; abstinence from sports utilizing the affected extremity; splinting; corticosteroid injection; and surgical decompression. Splinting and other conservative measures may be used; however, surgical decompression should not be deferred if symptoms persist more than six months. Decompression addresses the musculocutaneous nerve's course under the biceps tendon and the brachial fascia. Under direct observation a triangular window should be fashioned in the fascia. There should not be any fascial contact with the nerve regardless of the elbow's position. The best chance for nerve recovery and relief of symptoms occurs with early decompression.

REFERENCES

1. Bassett, F. H. and Nunley, A.J., *J. Bone Joint Surg.*, 64A, 1050, 1982.
2. Olson, I. A., *J. Anat.*, 105, 381, 1969.
3. Coyle, P. M., Nerve entrapment syndromes in the upper extremity, in *Principles of Orthopaedic Practice*, Dee, R., Ed., McGraw-Hill, New York, 1989.
4. Braddom, R. and Wolfe, C., *Arch. Phys. Med. Rehabil.*, 59, 290, 1978.

CARPAL TUNNEL SYNDROME

Compression of the median nerve occurs most commonly in a fibro-osseus canal on the palmar surface of the wrist, the carpal tunnel; the syndrome has been described frequently in the literature. In 1854, James Paget[1] first described chronic compression of the median nerve secondary to an old radius fracture at the level of the carpal tunnel. Others described disturbances ranging from vasomotor neurosis[2] to brachialgia paresthetica nocturia and from neurobrachialgia mechanica to acroparesthesia. These disturbances can be explained by Marie and Foix's[3] discussion in 1913, which implicated the transverse carpal ligament (flexor retinaculum) as the compressive agent. They described thenar atrophy due to median nerve compression which could be relieved by sectioning the ligament. While Moersch[4] and others used this approach, it was not until 1946 that Cannon and Love[5] published their results on nine patients. Due to the work of Brain, Wright, and Wilkinson[6] and Phalen[7] carpal tunnel surgery has become a refined and successful treatment of carpal tunnel syndrome.

ANATOMY

The median nerve courses through a fibro-osseus tunnel surrounded by the carpal bones, the transverse carpal ligament, and the flexor tendons. The scaphoid's and trapezium's tubercles bound the tunnel radially. The ulnar border consists of the pisiform and the hamate (Figure 1).

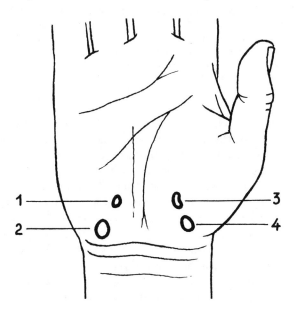

FIGURE 1.   Palpation can help identify the bony boundaries of the carpal tunnel.
1: Hook of the hamate; 2: pisiform bone; 3: tubercle of the trapezium; 4: tubercle of the scaphoid.

The inelastic transverse carpal ligament connects the radial and ulnar eminences of the wrist (Figure 2 a,b) and lies just below the skin. The ligament can course 2 to 5 cm longitudinally, 2 to 3 cm in width, and 0.5 cm in thickness. The tunnel itself narrows distally. The median nerve and tendons are relatively close to the ligament's posterior surface. The tendons of the flexor digitorum superficial (FDS) course above the tendons of the flexor digitorum profundus (FDP)

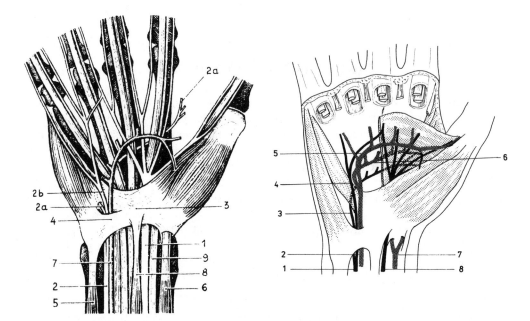

FIGURE 2a.   This figure reveals the detailed anatomy of the palm.

1: Median nerve; 2: ulnar nerve; 2a:deep branch (profundus) of the ulnar nerve; 2b: superficial branch of the ulnar nerve; 3: flexor retinaculum; 4: aponeurosis of the flexor carpi ulnaris muscle (tendinous end plate); 5: flexor carpi ulnaris muscle; 6: flexor carpi radialis muscle; 7: ulnar artery; 8: palmaris longus muscle; 9: flexor pollicis longus muscle.

FIGURE 2b.   This figure further delineates the vascular arcades.

1: Ulnar nerve; 2: ulnar artery; 3: deep branch of the ulnar nerve; 4: superficial branch of the ulnar nerve; 5: superficial palmar arterial arcade; 6: deep palmar arterial arcade; 7: radial artery; 8: median nerve.

and the flexor pollicis longus (FPL) (Figure 3). The FPL runs within its own synovial sheath — the radial digitocarpal sheath. The finger flexors run together in the ulnar digitocarpal sheath.

The median nerve lies superficial to the flexor tendons and remains the most sensitive to pressure of all the structures within the carpal tunnel. The anatomy of the median nerve and its branches varies so significantly that a cautious surgical approach is warranted to avoid a disabling sensory or motor deficit.[8] Before entering the tunnel, the median nerve gives off a palmar branch to supply the skin of the palm and thenar eminence. Within the tunnel, the median nerve may branch into a radial and ulnar component. The radial component supplies sensory branches to the palmar surfaces of the first and second fingers and motor branches to the abductor pollicis brevis, the opponens pollicis, and the superficial head of the flexor pollicis brevis. In 33% of individuals, the entire flexor pollicis brevis receives median nerve innervation. In 2% of the population, the adductor pollicis also receives median nerve innervation. Damage, whether surgical or compressive, leads to thenar atrophy and loss of abduction and opposition, as in an ape's hand. The ulnar component provides sensory branches to the palm surface of the second, third, and radial side of the fourth finger. Additionally, the median nerve can supply the dorsal surfaces of the second, third, and fourth fingers beyond the proximal interphalangeal joint. Patients commonly complain of sensory disturbances, pain, and cramps in these fingers. Spontaneous and provoked sensory disturbances, paresthesias, pain, and cramps commonly occur in these areas following Tinel's tests or hyperextension of the wrist.

Surgeons have performed extensive anatomical studies of the median nerve to improve surgical approaches and to decrease the risk of nerve injury (Table 1).[9,10] No simple approach exists. One must divide each layer and carefully examine for nerve branches. Unušić[11] recom-

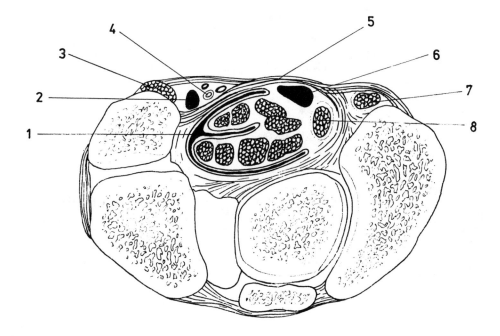

FIGURE 3.   This figure reveals the content of the carpal tunnel, which include nine tendons and the median nerve. Changes in the bony floor or ligamentous roof decrease the space available for the median nerve in the carpal tunnel. The ulnar nerve runs outside of the carpal tunnel.

1: Digitocarpal synovial invagination, ulnar side; 2: ulnar nerve; 3: flexor carpi ulnaris muscle; 4: ulnar artery; 5: flexor retinaculum or transverse carpal ligament; 6: median nerve; 7: flexor carpi radialis muscle; 8: flexor pollicis longus muscle.

mends exposure of the whole transverse ligament before release from the ulnar side. Papathanassiou[12] noted that motor branches may originate from the ulnar side of the ligament. Additionally, the smaller hand muscles may be fully innervated by either the median or ulnar nerve median as in the "all median hand" or "all ulnar hand" of Jušić and Šostarko.[13]

Etiology

Over 70 years ago, Marie and Foix[3] described several causes of carpal tunnel syndrome and suggested sectioning of the transverse carpal ligament. The success of surgical intervention underscores the mechanical nature of the syndrome.[5,14] The carpal tunnel represents a limited space containing bone, tendon, connective tissue, synovium, and nervous tissue. Therefore, diseases of or trauma to any of these components decreases the potential space and increases the pressure in the tunnel.[15-17] The median nerve, the most pressure sensitive component, manifests the disease's involvement of the wrist. Table 2 lists some of the literature describing pathological causes of carpal tunnel syndrome. This syndrome is three times more frequent in women than men and peaks between 30 and 50 years of age.

In order to use this information to guide surgical intervention, one would like to correlate disease states with their impact on connective tissue hypertrophy, synovial swelling, vascular supply (venous or arterial),[18-20] tissue edema, anatomic relationships, or general carpal tunnel pressure. Barnes and Currey[21] were unable to correlate synovial swelling on the palmar wrist surface with the appearance of carpal tunnel syndrome. Brain et al.[6] have investigated pressure variations in the carpal tunnel that range from 0 to 300 mm Hg depending on position. Chaise and Witovet[22] found that patients had a pressure of 25 mm Hg when a control group had a pressure of 4 to 6 mm Hg. With maximal extension and flexion, the control group had pressures of 30 mm Hg while the patients developed pressures up to 100 mm Hg. Brain et al.[6] suggested

TABLE 1
Variation of the Median Nerve

Author	Location	Innervation
Papathanassiou, 1968[12]	Ulnar origin of motor branch	Thenar motor
Kessler, 1969[62]	High division into ulnar and radial components	Hand
Linburg and Albright, 1970[10]	Ligament	Two motor branches, one pierces ligament
Ogden, 1972[63]	Forearm	Motor branch exits high, then merges with additional median nerve branch
Lanz, 1977[8]	Entire area of ligament	I. Variation of thenar nerve enervation
		II. Accessory braanch at distal portion
		III. High division
		IV. Accessory branch proximal to tunnel

that extension develops the biggest pressure. Other authors have duplicated these findings.[23] Leven and Huffman[24] found that conduction velocity was impaired most in positions of extreme flexion and extension. Thus, they recommended immobilization in a neutral position. Repetitive occupational tasks have currently come to the forefront in discussions of carpal tunnel syndrome.[6,25] Workers may spend a large portion of their time in flexion or extension placing their median nerve into prolonged high-pressure periods. Phalen[7] proposed that ischemia together with compression leads to the development of carpal tunnel syndrome.

CLINICAL SYMPTOMS AND SIGNS

As listed in Table 3, patients present with a constellation of symptoms and signs that depends on the duration of nerve compression.[26] Phalen[7] noted that 80% of patients present with sensory complaints. Spinner et al.[27] found that 100% of their patients had median paresthesias. These sensory complaints range from night pain that awakens the patient, to numbness and tingling in any of the sensory dermatomes of the median nerve. Since sensory fibers are more pressure sensitive than motor fibers, only 40% of patients will present initially with thenar hypotrophy or atrophy. Patients will complain of problems grasping or pinching.

Rheumatoid arthritis produces synovitis and intrinsic muscles atrophy in the hand. Synovitis can be seen causing asymmetric joint swelling. Komar[28] and Ford and Ali[29] discuss the two forms of carpal tunnel syndrome: acute and chronic. The acute form presents with severe pain, wrist or hand swelling, a cold hand, or decreased finger motion. Finger motion loss is due to a combination of pain and paresis. The chronic form presents with either a predominating sensory dysfunction or motor loss with trophic changes. Proximal pain in carpal tunnel syndrome may be present.[30]

TABLE 2
The Multitude of Etiologies for Carpal Tunnel Syndrome

Autoimmune/hematologic	Amyloidosis	Goldman, 1970
	Paraproteinemia	Huth et al.,, 1972
	Psoriasis	Shambaugh et al., 1974
	Sarcoidosis	
	Multiple myeloma	Swinton et al., 1970
	Lupus erythematous	Sidiq et al., 1972[64]
	Dermatomyositis	Quinones et al., 1966[65]
	Polyneuritis	Isaacs, 1972
	Blood dyscrasias	Blodget et al., 1962[66]
	Rheumatoid disease	Michaelis, 1950;[67] Smukler et al., 1963;[68] Brewerton, 1965; Phalen, 1966;[7] Barnes and Currey, 1967;[21] Phillips, 1967;[69] Androić, 1969;[70] Domljan, 1969;[50] Chamberlain and Bruckner, 1970; Bilić and Pećina, 1981, 1986;[37] Todorović and Smiljanić, 1982;[71] Conn, 1985; Moneim and Gribble, 1984[72]
	Hemophilia	Jabaley, 1978[77]
Congenital	Anatomical anomilies	Dekel and Coates, 1979;[73] Barfred and Ipsen, 1985;[74] Leslie and Ruby, 1985;[75] Asai et al., 1986[76]
Idiopathic	Primary tunnel stenosis essential	Dekel and Coates, 1979;[73] Brain et al., 1947;[6] Leven and Huffman, 1972;[24] Chaise and Witovët, 1984[22]
Infectious/inflammatory	Tenosynovitis	Phalen, 1966;[7]
	Tuberculosis	Mayer, 1964
Metabolic/hormonal	Pregnancy, menopause	Mletzko, 1962;[78] Tobin, 1967;[79] Ritland and Watson
	Oral contraceptives	Samour et al., 1972
	Diabetes mellitus	
	Renal failure/ dialysis	Allieu et al., 1983; [80] Benoit et al., 1988[81]
	Anticoagulant therapy	Hayden, 1964; Hartwell and Kurtay, 1966[42]
	Acromegaly/myxedema	Johnson and Shrewsbury, 1970;[82] Skanse, 1961[84]
Neoplasms	Nerve sheath tumors	
	Bone tumors/cysts	
	Ganglions	Seddon, 1952[84]

TABLE 2 (continued)
The Multitude of Etiologies for Carpal Tunnel Syndrome

	Neurofibromatosis	
	Metastatic disease	
Trauma	Fractures	Kaplan and Clayton, 1969
	Repetitive action, occupation induced	Wartmann, 1968; Hunt, 1909; Marti, 1960;[85] Masear et al., 1986[25]
	Degenerative joint disease	Nigst, 1981;[86] Leviet, et al., 1984[87]
	Pseudoarthrosis of the scaphoid	
Vascular	Circulatory disturbances	Baasch,1951;[88] Pećina, 1974;[16] Vainie, 1957[89]
	Reynaud's phenomenon	Ivković et al., 1976[18]

TABLE 3
Several Signs and Symptoms of Carpal Tunnel Syndrome

Sensory	Motor	Signs
Hypoesthesia	Hypotrophy	Trophic ulcers
	Weakness	Edema (21%)
Hypersthesias	Atrophy	
Numbness		
Burning		
Pain		
Night		
Stiffness		

Diagnosis and treatment of carpal tunnel syndrome must be prompt to avoid permanent nerve damage. Several basic clinical tests are available in the office. These tests seek to reproduce pain or paresthesias in the median nerve's distribution within 30 to 60 s of testing (Table 4). Tinel's sign[31] uses percussion over the transverse carpal ligament; Phalen's test uses maximal flexion of the wrist; and Wormser's test[32] (or reverse Phalen's) uses hyperextension of the wrist. Using the theory that compressed nerves are more sensitive to ischemia, Gilliatt and Wilson[33] and Wilson[34] introduced the use of a tourniquet to temporarily cut off the hand's arterial supply to the hand. Phalen[35] has found that 83% of his patients developed symptoms within 1 min. De la Caffiniere and Theis[36] found significant nerve damage if symptoms appeared in the first 15 s of tourniquet time. Bilić and Pećina[37] describes a sensitive pressure test that places digital pressure on the median nerve in the carpal tunnel while the patients place their entire extremity weight on their carpal tunnel. A tourniquet may be used in conjunction, but is not necessary. If symptoms appear after 10 s, the nerve's damage appears reversible. If paresthesias, hyperesthesia, or hypoesthesias appear in less than five seconds, the nerve's damage appears to be severe with low operative success. Bilić's pressure test may be modified and performed to assess other tunnel syndromes. Literature about other tests include Green's[38] description of the diagnostic and therapeutic value of carpal tunnel injection and Braun's[39] description of proactive testing in the diagnosis of dynamic carpal tunnel syndrome.

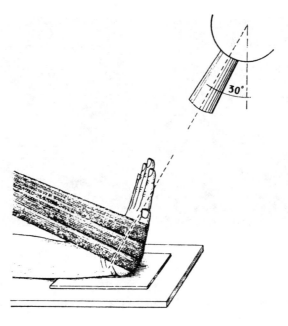

FIGURE 4.   Since the bony anatomy of the carpal tunnel may influence the development of the carpal tunnel syndrome, radiographic analysis of the carpal bones and arches complements the exam. Hart and Gaynov[90] and Barthold[43] proposed that a radiographic shot at 30° to an extended wrist would best visualize the carpal tunnel.

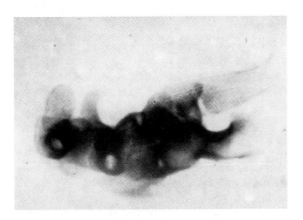

FIGURE 5A.   The result of a film shot as demonstrated in Figure 4.

While previously of limited value, radiographic studies of the carpal tunnel using magnetic resonance imaging (MRI) may yield an accurate anatomical assessment of the tunnel.[40] Hart and Gaynov,[41] Hartwell and Kurtay[42] and Barthold[43] describe axial X-rays of the hand in maximal dorsal flexion with the beam parallel to the fourth metacarpal bone and at 25 to 30° off a perpendicular line of the film (Figure 4). Figure 5 demonstrates the carpal tunnel with the hand in ulnar abduction. Mezgarzadeh et al.[44,45] described the anatomy of the tunnel as seen by MRI. Four general findings in carpal tunnel syndrome are described as follows: swelling of the median nerve; flattening of the median nerve; palmar bowing of the flexor retinaculum; and increased

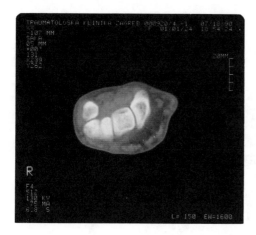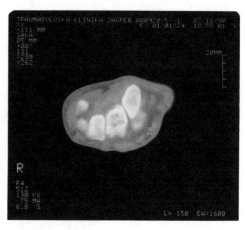

FIGURE 5B. A computerized tomogram of the carpal tunnel.

TABLE 4
Various Tests Used to Diagnose Carpal Tunnel Syndrome

Test	Findings	Sensitivity	Time	Prognosis
Tinel's	Paresthesias or pain	80%		
Phalen's	Paresthesias or pain	80%	Less than 1 min	
Wormser (Reverse Phalen)	Paresthesias or pain		Less than 1 min	
Tourniquet	Paresthesias or pain	83%	15 s	
Thenar atrophy	Decreased muscle bulk	36%		
Pressure test	Paresthesias		60 s if >10 s <5 s	
	Hyperesthesia			Not severe
	Hypoesthesia			Severe

signal intensity of the median nerve on T2-weighted images. Chen-Lung Liang[46] found that computed tomography (CT) images revealed sectional tunnel areas that were smaller than controls in idiopathic carpal tunnel syndrome, but were larger than controls in secondary carpal tunnel syndrome.

Before proceeding with surgery, one must eliminate any other causes of median nerve impairment prior to the carpal tunnel. Electromyographic studies bear an important role in differentiation among the possible affected areas.[47] The median nerve may be damaged from its roots in the cervical spine, through its division in the brachial plexus, or along its course in the arm. For example, involvement above the PT damages the palmaris branch whereas "below" at the CTS spares this branch. Vascular disease, toxic neuritis, and polyneuropathies may confuse the clinical picture. Radicular damage will present segmentally, whereas polyneuropathies will appear symmetrically or in areas of circulation. Characteristic electromyographic (EMG) findings in carpal tunnel syndrome are prolonged latency of motor impulses (more than four

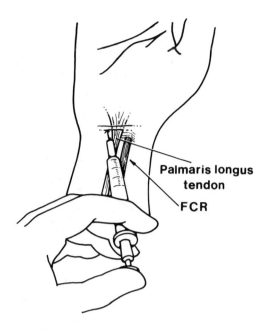

Palmaris longus
tendon

FCR

FIGURE 6.   Conservative therapy, which includes corticosteroid injection into the carpal
tunnel, may be tried within the framework of a
planned course of interventin. This figure illustrates the placement of the injection to allow entry
into the carpal tunnel.

milliseconds) and sensory impulses across the canal.[13,48] Even in the face of negative EMG findings, Phalen[35] felt that the diagnosis was warranted if the patient has sensory changes in the median nerve's distribution, position Tinel's and Phalan's tests, tenderness to pressure over the wrist, and hypotrophy of the thenar muscles.

TREATMENT

Treatment of carpal tunnel syndrome depends on the etiology, duration of symptoms, and intensity of nerve compression. If the syndrome is secondary to endocrine, hematologic, or other systemic diseases, the primary disease should be treated, with the surgeon following the reversal of median nerve compression. If this reversal does not occur or if the symptoms and signs progress, a treatment course should be followed.

Conservative therapy includes avoidance of trauma or repetitive actions, immobilization, anti-inflammatory medication, and corticosteroid injections (Figure 6). Duncan et al.[49] reported that in the U.S. 50 to 75% of all patients diagnosed with carpal tunnel syndrome have relief of symptoms without surgical treatment. The wrist is immobilized in the physiological position of slight extension with a dorsal splint for 3 to 6 weeks. While many patients have relief, the symptoms often recur. Corticosteroid injection into the canal may be offered to these patients.[50,51] Thin needle injections are placed into the carpal tunnel from the ulnar side of the palmaris longus tendon or the flexor carpi radialis tendon at an angle of 30° at the level of the proximal skin crease. The 30 to 50 mg of steroids (prednisone or similar steroid with or without an anesthetic agent) should not be injected into the nerve or tendons. Patients frequently suffer uneasiness, pain, and stiffness for 48 h as the additional fluid increases nerve compression in the tunnel. While injections may be repeated in 7 to 10 d to a total of 3 or 4 injections, failure to bring relief should be seen as an indication for surgical decompression. Prolonged conservative therapy trials of greater than 6 to 8 months can lead to less optimal results from surgery.[52] While

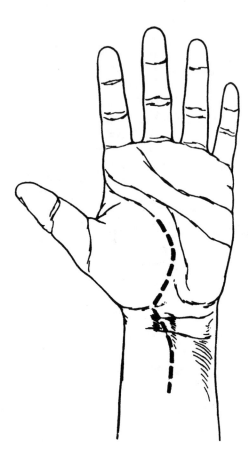

FIGURE 7.   There are many approaches to the carpal
tunnel, including a one-incision (classic), two-incision,
and arthroscropic approach to relieving compressio of
the median nerve. This figure shows the classic one-
incision approach, which stays ulnar to the thenar crease
and crosses the wrist crease obliquely.

results vary, Semple and Cargill[53] show a 97% success rate of symptoms persisting less than 6 months, and Hybbinette and Mannerfelt[54] show a 98% and a 90% success rate in relieving pain and sensory disturbances, respectively. Their studies described an objective improvement in motor symptoms.

Failure to respond within six months of conservative therapy or worsening of symptoms make surgical decompression necessary in spite of normal electromyography.[55] The carpal tunnel is approached paralleling the thenar crease to cross the palmar crease obliquely (Figure 7[11]). Care must be taken to preserve the palmaris branch of the median nerve.[56] While not uniformly present, the tendon of the palmaris longus muscle is identified and usually sectioned in older patients, but preserved in younger patients to maintain a tendon source for reconstructive procedures. The transverse carpal ligament or the flexor retinaculum can be approached from either the distal or proximal section as long as a constant watch is continued for the variable branches of the median nerve. The variations of the thenar branches alone range from numbers of branches to their points of departure from the carpal tunnel. The transverse carpal ligament must be fully released or partially removed to prevent recurrence of a tight fibrous band and thus the carpal tunnel syndrome.[57] Exploration of the median nerve usually reveals an hourglass deformity in the region of stenosis. A characteristic vascular blush is typically present. If these lesions cannot be found, a longitudinal incision is made in the epineurium. Neurolysis and tenosynovectomies remain controversial. Unušić[11] suggested microscopic interfascicular neurolysis while Curtis and Eversmann[58] recommend intrafascicular neurolysis when thenar atrophy or longstanding symptoms are present. Rheumatoid patients typically require synovectomies to decompress the area. This may require enlarging one's incision. Additionally, tendon function should be verified, since tendon damage or rupture is common in the rheumatoid population. Bilić and Pećina's review[37] found that surgery brought pain relief, improved function and esthetics features, and promoted deceleration of the disease process. Following decompression, the wrist should be dorsally splinted in extension and elevated for 24 to 48 h to reduce swelling. The time of immobilization varies from 1 to 3 weeks depending on the degree of exploration.

MacDonald et al.[59] describe the complications of surgical decompression as follows: recurrence of compression due to incomplete sectioning of the transverse carpal ligament; sympathetic dystrophy; trauma to the sensory or motor branches of the median nerve;[60] hypertrophic scar, palmar hematoma; flexor tendon prolapse; and adhesions limiting tendon function. These complications can be reduced by precise technique, postoperative care, and rehabilitation.[30,61]

While conservative measures may benefit some patients, the risks of prolonged compression combined with the high success rate of surgical decompression make a definite treatment schedule necessary. A definite treatment schedule will allow trials of conservative therapies prior to surgical decompression without exposing the patients to the risk of prolonged median nerve compression.

REFERENCES

1. Paget, J., Lectures on Surgical Pathology, Ed. 3, Ed. by Turner, W., Lindsay and Blakistan, 1865.
2. Rothnagel, 1867.
3. Marie, P. and Foix, Ch., *Rev. Neurol.,* 26, 647, 1913.
4. Moersch, F. P., *Proc. Staff. Meet. Mayo Clin.,* 13, 220, 1938.
5. Cannon, B. W. and Love, J. G., *Surgery,* 20, 210, 1946.
6. Brain ,W. P., Wright, A. D., and Wilkinson, M., *Lancet,* 1, 277, 1947.
7. Phalen, G. S., *J. Bone Joint Surg.,* 48A, 221, 1966.
8. Lanz, U., *J. Hand Surg.,* 2(1), 44, 1977.
9. Eiken, O., Carstam, N., and Eddeland, A., *Scand. J. Plast. Reconstr. Surg.,* 5, 149, 1971.
10. Linburg, R. M. and Albright, J. A., *J. Bone Joint Surg.,* 52A, 182, 1970.
11. Unušić, J.: *Izbor operatinog postupka kod sindroma karpalnog kanala,* disertacija, medicinski fakultet, Zagreb, 1981.
12. Pappathanassiou, B.T., *J. Bone Joint Surg.,* 50B, 156., 1968.
13. Jušić, A. and Šostarko, M., *Electromyogr. Clin. Neurophysiol.,* 13, 435, 1973.
14. Zachary, R. P., *Surg. Gynecol. Obst.,* 81, 213, 1945.
15. Krmpotić-Nemanić, J. and Pećina, M., *Treci simpozij o bolestima i ozljedama ßake,* Zagreb, 1972, str. 365.
16. Pećina, M., Cetvrti simpozij o bolestima i ozljedama ßake, Opatija, 1974, str. 203.
17. Pećina, M. and Bilić, R., Zbornik radova XII ortopedsko-traumatoloßkih dana Jugoslavije, Novi Sad, 1981, str. 175.
18. Ivković, T., Pećina, M., Rukavina, V., and Cuistović, F,: *Zbornik radova X orthopedsko-traumatoloßkih ana Jugoslavije,* Tjentißte, 1976, str. 472.
19. Rukavina, V., Pećina, M., Caustović, F., and Šoštarko, M., Peti simpozij o bolestima i ozljedama ßake, Dubrovnik, 1978, str. 15.
20. Ruszkowski, I. and Pećina, M., Drugi simpozij o bolestima i ozljedama ßake, Zagreb, 1970, str. 419.
21. Barnes, C. G. and Currey, H. L. F., *Ann. Rheum. Dis.,* 26, 226, 1967.
22. Chaise, F. and Witvoët, J., *Rev. Chir. Orthop.,* 70, 75, 1984.
23. Gelberman, R. H., Hergenroeder, P. T., Hargens, A. R., and Lundborg, G. N., Akeson, W. H., *J. Bone Joint Surg.,* 63A, 380, 1981.

24. Leven, B. and Huffmann, G., *Münch. Med. Wschr.*, 114, 1054, 1972.
25. Masear, V. R., Hayes, J. M., and Hyde, A. G., *J. Hand Surg.* [Am.], 11, 222, 1986.
26. Lister, G., *The Hand. Diagnosis and Indications,* Churchill Livingstone, Edinburg, 1984.
27. Spinner, J. R., Bachman, W. J., and Amadio, C. P., *Mayo Clin. Proc.,* 64, 829, 1989.
28. Komar, J., *Alagut-szindromak,* Medicina-Könyvkiako, Budapest, 1977.
29. Ford, D. J. and Ali, M.S., *J. Bone Joint Surg. [Br.],* 68, 758, 1986.
30. Das, S. K. and Brown, H. G., *Hand,* 8, 243, 1976.
31. Tinel, J., *Press Méd.,* 23, 388, 1915.
32. Wormser, P., *Fortsch. Neurol. Psych.,* 18, 211, 1950.
33. Gilliatt, R. W. and Wilson, T. G., *Lancet,* 2, 595, 1953.
34. Wilson, J. N., *J. Bone Joint Surg.,* 36A, 127, 1954.
35. Phalen, G. S., *Clin. Orthop.,* 83, 29, 1972.
36. de la Caffiniere, J. Y. and Theis, J. C., *Rev. Chir. Orthop.,* 70, 245, 1984.
37. Bilić, R. and Pećina, M., *Acta Orthop. Lugosl.,* 17(3), 191, 1986.
38. Green, D. P., *J. Hand Surg. [Am.],* 9, 850, 1984.
39. Braun, R. M., Davidson, K., and Doehr, S., *J. Hand Surg. [Am.],* 14, 195, 1989.
40. Schober, R. and Bayard, C. A., *Fortsch. Rontg.,* 90, 266, 1959.
41. Hart, V. L. and Gaynov, V., *J. Bone Joint Surg.,* 23, 382, 1941.
42. Hartwell and Kurtay, 1966.
43. Barthold, G., *Zentralbl. Chir.,* 17, 696, 1960.
44. Mezgarzadeh, M., Schneck, D. C., and Bonakdarpour, A., *Radiology,* 171, 743, 1989.
45. Mezgarzadeh, M., Schneck, D. C., and Bonakdarpour, A., *Radiology,* 171, 749, 1989.
46. Chen-Lung Liang, *J. Jpn. Orthop. Assoc.,* 61, 1033, 1987.
47. Melvin, J. L., Schushmann, J. A., and Lanese, R. R., *Arch. Phys. Med. Rehabil.,* 54, 69, 1973.
48. Sprindler, H. A. and Dellon, A. L., *J. Hand Surg.,* 7, 260, 1982.
49. Duncan, K. H., Lewis, R. C., Jr., Foreman, K. A., Nordyke, M. D., *J. Hand Surg. [Am.],* 12, 384, 1987.
50. Domljan, Z., *Lijec. Vjesn.,* 91, 959, 1969.
51. Flatt, A. E., *The Case of the Rheumatoid Hand,* C. V. Mosby, St. Louis, 1974.
52. Schink, W. and Spier, W., *Wiedenrherst. Chir. Traumat.,* 9, 8, 1967.
53. Semple, J. C. and Cargill, A. O., *Lancet,* 3, 918, 1969.
54. Hybbinette, C. G. and Mannerfelt, L., *Acta Orthop. Scand.,* 46, 610, 1975.
55. Grundberg, A. B., *J. Hand Surg.,* 8, 348, 1983.
56. Rowland, S. A., *Clin. Orthop.,* 103, 89, 1974.
57. Wulle, C., *Ann. Chir. Main,* 6, 203, 1987.
58. Curtis, R. M. and Eversmann, W. W., *J. Bone Joint Surg.,* 55A, 733, 1973.
59. MacDonald, R. I., Lichtman, D. M., Hanlon, J. J., and Wilson, J. N., *J. Hand Surg.,* 3, 70, 1978.
60. Lily, C. J. and Magell, T. D., *J. Hand Surg.,* 10A, 399, 1985.
61. Inglis, A. E., *J. Bone Joint Surg.,* 62A, 1208, 1980.
62. Kessler, I., *Clin. Orthop.,* 67, 124, 1969.
63. Ogden, J. A., *J. Bone Joint Surg.,* 54A, 1779, 1972.
64. Sidiq, M., Kirsner, A. B., and Sheon, R. P., *JAMA,* 222, 1416, 1972.
65. Quinones, C. A., Perry, H. O., and Rushton, J. C., *Arch. Dermatol.,* 94, 20, 1966.
66. Blodget, R. C., Lipscomb, P. R., and Hill, R. W., *JAMA,* 182, 814, 1962.
67. Michaelis, L. S., *Proc. R. Soc. Med.,* 43, 414, 1950.
68. Smukler, N. M., Patterson, J. R., Lorenz, H., and Weiner, L., *Arthritis Rheum.,* 6, 298, 1963.
69. Phillips, R. S., *Ann. Rheum. Dis.,* 26, 59, 1967.
70. Androić, S., *Reumatizam,* 94, 109, 1969.
71. Todorović, N. and Smiljanić, P., *Med. Jan.,* 14(2-4), 215, 1982.
72. Moneim, M. S. and Gribble, T. J., *J. Hand Surg.,* 9, 580, 1984.
73. Dekel, S. and Coates, R., *Lancet,* 2, 1024, 1979.
74. Barfred, T. and Ipsen, T., *J. Hand Surg. [Am.],* 10, 246, 1985.
75. Leslie, B. M. and Ruby L.K., *Orthopedics,* 8, 1165, 1985.
76. Asai, M., Wong, A. C. W., Matsuanga, T., and Akahoshi, Y., *J. Hand Surg. [Am.],* 11, 218, 1986.
77. Jabaley, M. E., *Hand Surg.,* 3(1), 82, 1978.
78. Mletzko, J., *Chirurg.,* 33, 414, 1962.
79. Tobin, S. M., *Am. J. Obstet. Gynecol.,* 97, 493, 1967.
80. Allieu, Y., Asencio, G., Mailhe, D. Baldet, P., and Mion, C., *Rev. Chir. Orthop.,* 69, 233, 1983.
81. Benoit, J., Guiziou, B., Godinger, J. J., Delons, S., and Got, Cl., *Rev. Chir. Orthop.* (Suppl. II), 74, 162, 1988.
82. Johnson, R. K. and Shrewsbury, M. M., *J. Bone Joint Surg.,* 52A, 269, 1970.
83. Skanse, B., *Acta Chir. Scand.,* 121, 476, 1961.
84. Seddon, H. J., *J. Bone Joint Surg.,* 34B, 386, 1952.

85. Marti, R., *Schw. Med. Wochensch.,* 35, 986, 1960.
86. Nigst, H., *Ther. Unsch.,* 38, 1208, 1981.
87. Leviet, D., Ebelin, M., Meriaux, J. L., and Vilain, R., *Rev. Chir. Orthop.,* 70, 79, 1984.
88. Baasch, E., *Schw. Arch. Neurol. Neurochir. Psych.,* 67, 443, 1951.
89. Vainie, K., *Acta Rheum. Scand.,* 4, 22, 1957.
90. Hart, V. L. and Gaynov, V., *Radiol. Clin. Phot.,* 18, 23, 1942.

ULNAR TUNNEL SYNDROME
(GUYON'S CANAL SYNDROME)

Analogous to median nerve compression at the wrist, ulnar nerve compression at the wrist occurs in Guyon's canal, producing the ulnar tunnel syndrome. Guyon,[1] a French surgeon, described the fibro-osseus tunnel shown in Figures 2 and 3 of Chapter 13. While not as common as carpal tunnel syndrome, ulnar tunnel syndrome should be suspected and a detailed physical exam performed in all patients complaining of hand numbness.

ANATOMY

The ulnar tunnel or Guyon's canal lies at the level of the proximal carpal bones along the ulnar border. The transverse carpal ligament forms the floor of the tunnel with the tendinous insertion of the flexor carpi ulnaris muscle forming the roof. The ulnar and radial borders consist of the pisiform and hamate bones, respectively. Triangular in shape, as seen in Figure 1, the tunnel narrows from a large volar base to a dorsal point. Anatomical studies have found the tunnel's height to range from 8 to 15 mm.

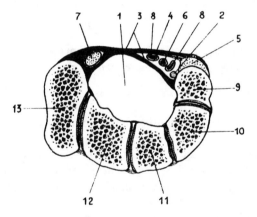

FIGURE 1.   While not at risk from compression in carpal tunnel syndrome, the ulnar nerve does not run in its own tunnel with the inherent risks of compression when pathology affects the tunnel's components.

1: Carpal tunnel; 2: ulnar nerve; 3: flexor retinaculum; 4: aponeurosis of the flexor carpi ulnaris muscle (tendinous insertion); 5: flexor carpi ulnaris muscle; 6: ulnar artery; 7: flexor carpi radialis muscle; 8: ulnar veins; 9: pisiform; 10: triquetrium; 11: hamate; 12: capinate; 13: scaphoid (navicular).

Blood vessels and the palmar branch of the ulnar nerve pass through the tunnel. Proximal to entering the canal, the ulnar nerve divides into a dorsal branch and a palmar branch that further divides into a superficial and a deep branch prior to the tunnel (Figure 2 of Chapter 13). Only the superficial and deep palmar branches of the ulnar nerve run in the ulnar tunnel. Therefore, the dorsal branch is spared in the ulnar tunnel syndrome, while it is affected in the ulnar nerve compression in the ulnar sulcus behind the medial epicondyle. The superficial branch of the palmar branch innervates the palmaris brevis muscle, the palmar skin of the fifth finger, and the ulnar skin of the fourth finger. The deep branch innervates the hypothenar muscles, the two lateral lumbricals, all the interossei muscles, the adductor pollicis muscle, and the deep head of

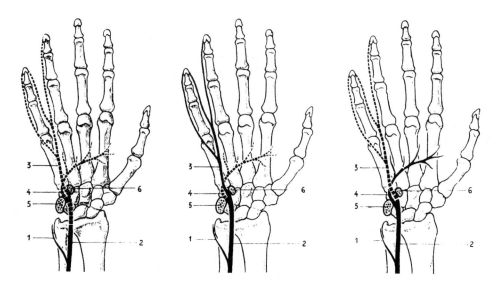

FIGURE 2.   This figure indicates the various forms of ulnar nerve compression and the branches affected.
1: Dorsal branch of the ulnar nerve; 2: ulnar nerve; 3: superficial branch of the ulnar nerve; 4: deep (profundus)
branch of the ulnar nerve; 5: pisiform; 6: hook of the hamate.

the flexor pollicis brevis muscle. Therefore, compression of the superficial branch yields mixed motor and sensory symptoms, while compression of the deep branch yields only motor symptoms.

ETIOLOGY

Shea and McClain[2] describe three different types of ulnar nerve compression in the ulnar tunnel or Guyon's canal based on motor and sensory disturbances. As shown in Figure 2, the compression occurs in the tunnel and produces symptoms distal to the compression, depending on which branches are compromised. The first type of compression can also be known as the "upper form", since the compression occurs quite proximally and prevents any ulnar nerve innervation. Mumenthaler's sign will be positive since resisted fifth-finger abduction will not create palmar creases because the palmaris brevis does not function. The second type of compression produces only motor dysfunction. Therefore, only the deep branch is compromised. The "middle form" infers compression prior to the hypothenar muscle branches. The "lower form" of the second type infers deep-branch compression distal to the hypothenar muscle branch thereby, sparing it. The third form of compression has predominately sensory symptoms, since the superficial branch is compromised, affecting the dermatome as shown in Figure 2. We disagree with the sign associated with the upper form, since a lesion in this area should knock out all motor function in the hand that is due to the ulnar nerve.

There are multiple etiologies of mechanical irritation and damage to the nerve in the ulnar tunnel.[3] Post-traumatic compression and anatomical anomalies represent some of the more common etiologies. Trauma may come from events as different as fractures of the hook of the hamate[4] or riding bicycles.[5] In war time, German soldiers rode bicycles over long distances leading to nerve compression from the handlebars that was described in the literature as *Radfahrerlähung*. Anomalies may include the passage of the fourth-finger flexor tendon through the tunnel. Ganglions, typically arising from degenerative arthritis, are present in 28.7% of patients with compressive symptoms. Occupationally related external compression,[6,7] vascular disturbances, pisotriquetral joint arthritis,[8-10] bursitis of a bursa near the pisiform bone,[11] giant cell tumor of tendon sheath,[12] inflammatory diseases (including rheumatic diseases), edema,[13] aberrant muscles,[14-16] and idiopathic cases complete the list of proposed etiologies. Ulnar artery

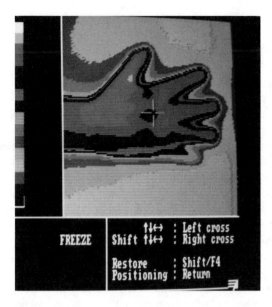

FIGURE 3.   Thermographic "amputation" of the ulnar sides of the fourth and fifth fingers in a patient with ulnar tunnel syndrome (syndrome of Guyon's canal).

aneurysms[17] or thromboangiitis[18] may produce the syndrome. Included in the category of muscular disturbances leading to compression is hypertrophy of the flexor carpi ulnaris muscle.[19]

CLINICAL SIGNS AND SYMPTOMS

While hypothenar atrophy may not be present, patients describe uncertainty in their hand movements, including grasping. Pain may arise early and be aggravated by wrist extension. Numbness, tingling, and paresthesias may be found in the appropriate distribution. Worse at night, this involvement of the third, fourth, and fifth fingers may force patients to stop using the hand. Forced palmar (Phalen's sign) and dorsal flexion (Wormser's or reverse Phalen's sign) cause paresthesias in the fourth and fifth fingers, with occasional involvement of the second and third fingers.[20,21] Adduction of the fifth finger and abduction and adduction of the thumb and other fingers is not impaired (a fact important for differential diagnosis). Tests used to elicit symptoms in carpal tunnel syndrome are also used to evaluate ulnar tunnel syndrome. Pressure and tapping on the carpal tunnel may produce paresthesias in the palmar branch of the ulnar nerve's dermatome. Use of a blood pressure cuff to induce ischemia may reproduce pain and paresthesias within minutes that may spread proximally and persist after cuff release. Late signs of compression are hypotrophy and atrophy leading to cramps and grasp weakness.

Other studies are available to identify compression in the ulnar tunnel. Hart and Gaynov[22] and Barthold[23] recommended special radiographic axial views of the carpal tunnel to evaluate abnormal configurations. Electromyographic and conduction velocity studies can help identify the level of nerve dysfunction.[24] Thermography can also be used in diagnosis of ulnar tunnel syndrome (Figure 3). Additionally, the presence of a coexisting carpal tunnel syndrome may be appreciated allowing both neuropathies to be treated simultaneously.[25] Laboratory examinations will allow rheumatologic diseases to be identified to optimize treatment.[26,27] While positive tests support one's clinical diagnosis, negative or borderline negative results must be kept in perspective, and anomalous innervation must be kept in mind.[28]

TREATMENT

Conservative therapy remains the first line in treating ulnar nerve compression in the ulnar tunnel or Guyon's Canal. Trials of conservative therapies should not be continued indefinitely, since prolonged compression may lead to permanent nerve damage. While conservative therapy may take up to 6 months to work, absence of relief by 6 months should be surgically treated without delay. Avoidance of repetitive trauma, rest immobilization (splinting), local corticosteroid injection, and anti-inflammatory medication may be tried individually and in combination to achieve relief. Any underlying diseases leading to nerve damage must be treated.

Muscle atrophy or hypotrophy, persistent symptoms (past 6 months), or failure of conservative therapy to bring permanent relief indicates patients with severe neurological deficits. These patients require surgical decompression with complete neurolysis of both the motor and sensory branches.[29,30] The approach to the tunnel removes the tendinous floor including the transverse carpal ligament (flexor retinaculum). The tunnel is cleared and adhesions removed. The nerve below the tendinous arch of the hypothenar muscles must also be released. Following surgery, patients are immobilized in splints for ten days to two weeks before therapy begins. Surgical results will be poorer when definitive therapy is postponed or when the patient is older than 65 years of age.

While less common, ulnar tunnel syndrome may occur in conjunction with carpal tunnel syndrome. Therefore, one must assess the status of the median nerve before proceeding to ulnar tunnel release. Wissinger[31] described a limited approach to both tunnels. If involved, the median nerve should be released.

REFERENCES

1. Guyon, F., *Bull. Soc. Anat. Paris,* 6, 184, 1861.
2. Shea, J. D. and McClain, E. J., *J. Bone Joint Surg.,* 51A, 1095, 1969.
3. Souquet, R. and Mansat, M., Syndrome du canal de Guyon, in *Syndromes Canalaires du Membre Supérieur,* Souquet, R., Ed., Expansion Scientifique Francaise, Paris, 1983.
4. Torisu, T., *Clin. Orthop.,* 83, 91, 1972.
5. Eckman, P. B., Perlstein, G., and Altrocchi, P. H., *Arch. Neurol.,* 32, 130, 1975.
6. Hunt, J. R., *J. Nerv. Ment. Dis.,* 35, 637, 1908.
7. Pecina, M. and Grospic, R., *Riv. Patol. Aparato Locom.,* 1, 183, 1981.
8. Jenkins, S. A., *J. Bone Joint Surg.,* 33B, 532, 1951.
9. Carrol, R. E. and Green, D. P., *Clin. Orthop.,* 83, 24, 1972.
10. Carrol, R. E. and Coyle, M. P., *J. Hand Surg.,* 10A, 703, 1985.
11. Seddon, H. J., *J. Bone Joint Surg.,* 34B, 386, 1952.
12. Hayes, J. R., Mulholland, R. C., and O'Conner, B. T., *J. Bone Joint Surg.,* 51B, 469, 1969.
18. Leslie, I. E., *Hand,* 12, 271, 1980.
14. Jeffery, A. K., *J. Bone Joint Surg.,* 53B, 718, 1971.
15. Swanson, A. B., Biddulph, S. L., Baughman, F. A., and De Groot, G., *Clin. Orthop.,* 83, 64, 1972.
16. Turner, M. S. and Caird, D. M., *Hand,* 9, 140, 1977.
17. Nade, S., *Injury,* 3, 169, 1972.
18. Dupont, C., Cloutier, G. E., Prevost, Y., and Dion, M. A., *J. Bone Joint Surg.,* 47A, 757, 1965.
19. Harrelson, J. M. and Newman, M., *J. Bone Joint Surg.,* 57A, 554, 1975.
20. Wormser, P., *Fortsch. Neurol. Psych.,* 18, 211, 1950.
21. Phalen, G. S., *J. Bone Joint Surg.,* 48A, 221, 1966.
22. Hart, V. L. and Gaynov, V., *J. Bone Joint Surg.,* 23, 382, 1941.
23. Barthold, G., *Zentralbl. Chir.,* 17, 696, 1960.
24. Jušić, A., *Reumatizam,* 16, 141, 1969.
25. Ruszkowski, I. and Pecina, M., *Lijec. Vjesn.,* 92, 781, 1970.
26. Androić, S., *Reumatizam,* 94, 109, 1969.
27. Domljan, Z., *Lijec. Vjesn.,* 91, 959, 1969.
28. Mannerfelt, L., *Acta Orthop. Scand.,* Suppl. 87, 1966.
29. Kleinert, H. E. and Hayes, J. E., *Plast. Reconstr. Surg.,* 47, 21, 1971.

30. Grundberg, A. B., *J. Hand Surg.*, 9B, 72, 1984.
31. Wissinger, H. A., *Plast. Reconstr. Surg.*, 56, 501, 1975.

SYNDROME OF THE DEEP BRANCH OF THE ULNAR NERVE
(THE PISO-HAMATE HIATUS SYNDROME)

The deep branch of the ulnar nerve risks compression as it passes through a fibro-osseus tunnel formed by the tendinous origin of the hypothenar muscles (Figure 1). While similar to ulnar nerve compression in Guyon's tunnel if only the motor branch is compressed, the syndrome of the deep branch of the ulnar nerve, known to Uruburu et al.[1] as the *piso-hamate hiatus syndrome,* does not affect the abductor digiti minimi muscle, whose branch originates before the tendinous arch. Therefore, at times this syndrome can be known as the *syndrome of the tendinous arch of the hypothenar muscle.*

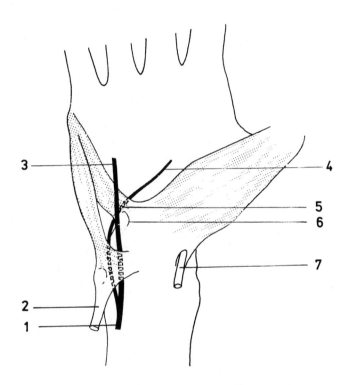

FIGURE 1.   This figure shows the anatomy along the hypothenar area of the palm..
1: Ulnar nerve; 2: flexor carpi ulnaris muscle; 3: superficial branch of the ulnar nerve; 4: deep branch of the ulnar nerve; 5: tendinous origin of the hypothenar muscles; 6: tendinous arch of the hypothenar muscles; 7: flexor carpi radialis muscle.

ANATOMY

The fibro-osseus tunnel in the region of the hypothenar muscles has two bony walls and two fibrous walls. The ulnar and radial walls consist of the pisiform bone and the hamate bones, respectively. Both the piso-hamate ligament that spans the floor and the tendinous arch that forms the roof have been implicated in nerve compression. Through cadaver studies, Hayes et al.[2] emphasized the importance of the piso-hamate ligament in ulnar nerve compression. Connecting the pisiform and the hook of the hamate bone, the tendinous arch serves as the origin for some of the hypothenar muscles: the adductor digiti minimi, flexor digiti minimi brevis, and the opponens digiti minimi muscles.

The deep branch of the ulnar nerve passes through this tunnel and gives motor fibers to the hypothenar muscles except the palmaris brevis muscle, which receives its innervation from the superficial branch. In addition, the interossei muscles, the two ulnar lumbrical muscles, the adductor pollicis muscle, and the deep head of the flexor pollicis brevis muscle receive innervation from the deep branch of the ulnar nerve. Sparing of the abductor digiti minimi muscle, whose motor branch originates proximal to the tunnel, allows differentiation of this syndrome from ulnar nerve compression proximally (i.e., Guyon's Tunnel in ulnar tunnel syndrome).[3]

ETIOLOGY

While having some similar etiologies to those causing ulnar tunnel compression,[4] compression of the deep branch of the ulnar nerve occurs most frequently with ganglion cysts.[2,5] It also occurs with anomalous muscles,[6] intraneural cysts,[7] carpal bone fractures including hamate fractures[8] ulnar artery anomalies and diseases,[9] and chronic wrist trauma.[10,11] including occupational neuritis.[12]

CLINICAL SYMPTOMS AND SIGNS

Patients present with poorly localized pain in the innervation field of the deep branch of the ulnar nerve. Since the deep branch has no sensory component, the patients do not have paresthesias or hypesthesias. In this syndrome, the palmaris brevis and abductor digiti minimi muscles typically continue to function, in contrast to ulnar tunnel syndrome, since their innervation originates proximal to the tendinous arch but distal to the ulnar tunnel. Since deep-branch compression presents with motor signs, the differential diagnosis must include the second type of ulnar tunnel syndrome, progressive spinal muscle atrophy, and lateral amyotrophic sclerosis. Electromyographic studies play an important role in localizing the lesion.

TREATMENT

Conservative therapy consists of avoidance of repetitive wrist trauma, short-term immobilization, and anti-inflammatory medication; and local corticosteroid injections should precede surgical decompression. Surgical release of the tendinous arch, from which the hypothenar muscles take their origin, is usually sufficient for decompression.

REFERENCES

1. Uriburu, T. J. F., Morchio, F. J., and Marin, J. C., *J. Bone Joint Surg.,* 58A, 145, 1976.
2. Hayes, J. R., Mulholland, R. C., and O'Conner, B. T., *J. Bone Joint Surg.,* 51B, 469, 1969.
3. Pecina, M. and Bilic, R., Zbornik radova XII ortopedsko-traumatoloskih dana Jugoslavije, Novi Sad, 1981, 175.
4. Shea, J. D. and McClain, E. J., *J. Bone Joint Surg.,* 51A, 1095, 1969.
5. Seddon, H. J., *J. Bone Joint Surg.,* 34B, 386, 1952.
6. Schielderup, H., *J. Bone Joint Surg.,* 46B, 361, 1964.
7. Bowers, W. H. and Doppelt, S. M., *J. Bone Joint Surg.,* 61A, 612, 1979.
8. Harvard, F. M., *J. Bone Joint Surg.,* 43, 1197, 1961.
9. Millender, J. H., Nalehoff, E. A., and Kasden, E., *Arch. Surg.,* 105, 686, 1977.
10. Bakle, J. L. and Waff, M. G., *Arch. Neurol. Psych.,* 60, 549, 1948.
11. Domljan, Z., *Lijec. Vjesn.,* 91, 959, 1969.
12. Hunt, J. R., *J. Nerv. Ment. Dis.,* 35, 637, 1908.

SYNDROME OF THE TENDINOUS ARCH
OF THE ADDUCTOR POLLICIS MUSCLE
(SYNDROME OF THE TERMINAL PART
OF THE DEEP BRANCH OF THE ULNAR NERVE)

The syndrome of the tendinous arch of the adductor pollicis muscle occurs when the terminal portion of the deep branch of the ulnar nerve gets compressed between the tendinous arch connecting the transverse and oblique heads of the adductor pollicis muscle (Figure 1).

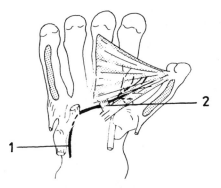

FIGURE 1.   As the deep branch of the ulnar nerve (1) transverses the palm, it may be compressed under the tendinous arch (2) connecting the oblique and transverse heads of the adductor pollicis muscle.

ANATOMY

The transverse head of the adductor pollicis muscle originates from the anterior margin of the third metacarpal bone. The oblique head and the deep head of the flexor pollicis brevis muscle share a common origin, the ligaments covering the trapezoid and the capitate carpal bones. Connecting the heads of the two adductor pollicis, the tendinous arch forms the roof of a tunnel whose floor is the third metacarpal bone. The terminal branch of the deep branch of the ulnar nerve dives through this tunnel to innervate the adductor pollicis.

ETIOLOGY

Repetitive trauma to the midpalm may lead to the development of this syndrome. This type of trauma is common in professions that require prolonged gripping activities and in sports like cycling. Flat rectangular grips may be worse offenders than round handles.[1] Fractures, tumors, or any disease that affects the third metacarpal bone may elevate the floor, narrow the tunnel, and lead to nerve compression.[2-4]

CLINICAL SYMPTOMS AND SIGNS

Patients may present with blunt midpalmar pain without paresthesias, isolated weakness, and atrophy of the adductor pollicis muscle. Pressure at the base of the third metacarpal bone may reproduce pain. Electromyographic analysis shows that conduction time is prolonged for the adductor pollicis muscle but not for other hypothenar muscles.

TREATMENT
Treatment consists in removal of the cause by conservative methods. Local injection of corticosteroids usually relieves the compression;[5] however, abnormalities of the tunnel's bony structure may necessitate a surgical therapy.

REFERENCES
1. Boëda, A. G., Pesque, F., and Hillmeyer, J. C., *Méd. Sport,* 47, 9, 1973.
2. Commandre, F., *Pathologie Abarticulaire,* Laboratoire Cétrane, Paris, 1977.
3. Domljan, Z., *Lijec. Vjesn.,* 91, 959, 1969.
4. Pecina, M. and Bilic, R., Zbornik radova XII ortopedsko-traumatoloßkih dana Jugoslavije, Novi Sad, 1981, pp. 175.
5. Serre, H., Simon, L., and Claustre, I., *Rev. Rheumat.,* 33, 231, 1966.

SYNDROME OF THE SUPERFICIAL BRANCH OF THE RADIAL NERVE
(CHEIRALGIA PARESTHETICA)

Making an analogy to paresthetic meralgia, Wartenberg in 1932[1] suggested the name *cheirlagia paresthetica* to define isolated neuropathy of the superficial branch of the radial nerve. Also known as Wartenberg's disease, radial nerve compression can occur throughout its course in the forearm, especially in the tunnel region beneath the tendon of the brachioradialis muscle. The work of Schlesinger,[2] Stopford,[3] and Matzdorff[4] helped Wartenberg[1] clarify the syndrome. Sprofkin,[5] Wartenberg,[6] and Bora and Osterman[7] suggested that cheiralgia paresthesia was less rare than originally almost thought.

ANATOMY

The superficial ramus or branch divides from the radial nerve as it lies in the radial cubital sulcus. As shown in Figure 1, this branch travels distally over the supinator muscle and the pronator teres. Passing over the pronator teres muscle, the nerve dips under the ulnar border of the brachioradialis muscle and bends dorsally to run along the radius. The superficial branch, at a point between the middle and distal thirds of the radius, arches dorsally through a tunnel in the antebrachial fascia to terminate in the skin beyond the radial styloid. The dorsal digital nerves, the terminal branches of the superficial branch, supply sensation to the dorsal skin of the first, second, and radial side of the third digits to the base of the second phalanx. As skin dermatomes overlap, the only autonomous region of the superficial radial nerve is the dorsal web space closest to the thumb.

ETIOLOGY

While predominantly injured by trauma to the radius, the superficial branch of the radial nerve can be injured by multiple reported causes as follows: surgical trauma (especially during operations for De Quervain's disease) or other trauma to the wrist,[8,9] compressive plaster casts, intravenous infusion in the forearm and wrist, osteoarthritic changes of the wrist, and chronic irritation from tight cuffs or watch straps.[3,10-13] This list leaves many cases unexplained except by dynamic relationships of the nerve and brachioradialis tendon near the radius.

CLINICAL SYMPTOMS AND SIGNS

Characteristically, patients present with paresthesias without weakness or atrophy. Burning pain, sensory changes, and night pain are appreciated along the dorsal wrist, thumb, and web space (Figure 2). The simple irritation of clothing in this region may be enough to produce paresthesias. One will generally find a positive Tinel's test. Chronic cases will present with trophic skin changes evident by the skin's shiny thin surface and lack of hair. To differentiate cheiralgia paresthetica from a cervical radiculopathy, one only needs to note that there are no motor signs nor any affect on other areas of radicular involvement.

TREATMENT

Damage to the radial nerve can lead to disability, especially if the patient's dominant hand is involved. Therefore, extreme caution must be exercised when dissecting proximal to the base of the thumb and near the brachioradialis tendon. If the syndrome occurs from external compression, conservative therapy can be successful. Local application of corticosteroids, anesthetic creams, histamine, and ionophoresis may yield some results. Surgical exploration may be necessary if conservative therapy fails.[12,14] If the nerve is trapped by scar tissue, release, neurolysis, and coverage with healthy tissue should be performed. The presence of a neuroma

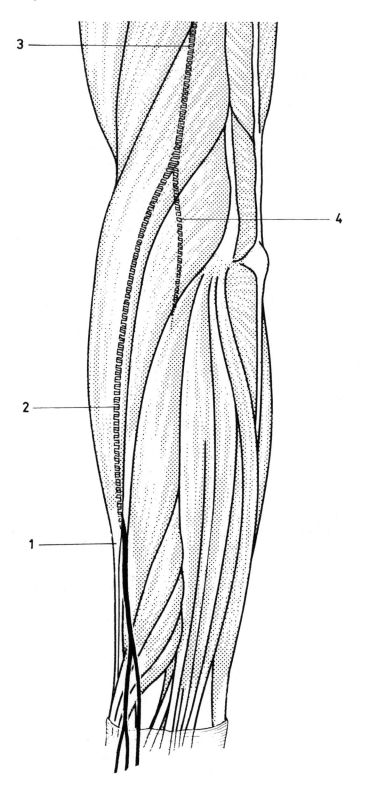

FIGURE 1.   This figure charts the course of the radial nerve in the forearm.
1: Brachioradialis muscle; 2: superficial branch of the radial nerve; 3: radial nerve 4:
deep branch of the radial nerve.

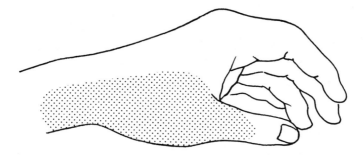

FIGURE 2.   This figure illustrates the region of the forearm supplied by the superficial branch of the radial nerve. Nerve compression in this area leads to paresthesias consisting of burning pain, commonly known as cheiralgia paresthetica.

produces a guarded prognosis for recovery and relief.[15] Hypesthesia due to nerve resection may be acceptable when faced with continued burning pains and paresthesias. However, the loss of hand sensation will disable a patient and increase the risk of injury even in daily activities.

REFERENCES

1. Wartenberg, R., *Zach. Neurol. Psych.*, 141, 145, 1932.
2. Schlesinger, H., *Neurologisches Centralblatt.*, 30, 1218, 1911.
3. Stopford, J. S. B., *Lancet*, 1, 993, 1922.
4. Matzdorff, P., *Klin. Wchs.*, 5, 1187, 1926.
5. Sprofkin, B. E., *Neurology*, 4, 857, 1954.
6. Wartenberg, R., *Neurology*, 4, 106, 1954.
7. Bora, F. W. and Osterman, A. L., *Clin. Orthop.*, 163, 20, 1982.
8. Linscheid, R. L., *Arch. Surg.*, 91, 942, 1965.
9. Griffiths, J. C., *Br. Med. J.*, 2, 277, 1966.
10. Dorfman, L. J. and Jaepram, P., *JAMA*, 239, 957, 1958.
11. Bierman, H. R., *N. Engl. J. Med.*, 261, 237, 1959.
12. Braidwood, A. S., *J. Bone Joint Surg.*, 57B, 380, 1975.
13. Pecina, M. and Bilic, R., *Zbornik radova XII ortopedsko-traumatoloßkih dana Jugoslavije*, Novi Sad, 1981, pp. 175.
14. Dellon, A. L. and Mackinnon, S. E., *J. Hand Surg.*, 11A, 199, 1986.
15. Coyle, P. M., Nerve entrapment syndromes in the upper extremity, in *Principles of Orthopaedic Practice*, Dee, R., Ed., McGraw-Hill, New York, 1989.

COLLATERAL DIGITAL NERVE SYNDROME

The terminal branches of the median and the ulnar nerves can be compressed in the region of the metacarpophalangeal joints resulting in pain and paresthesias in the corresponding digits. The terminal nerve branches supply only sensory innervation to the skin and joints of the fingers. Therefore, signs of sensory dysfunction indicate nerve compression.

ANATOMY

The heads of the second to the fifth metacarpal bones near the metacarpophalangeal joints are connected by superficial and deep transverse metacarpal ligaments. These ligaments form metacarpal tunnels through which pass the digital nerves, the common palmar digital arteries and veins, and the tendons of the lumbrical muscles (Figure 1). The digitorum palmaris communis nerves, the branches of the ulnar and the median nerves, branch before or within the tunnels to provide terminal branches (the digitorum palmaris proprius nerves) to neighboring surfaces of corresponding fingers. The lumbricals receive their innervation from branches proximal to the tunnels. The third digital branch, a branch of the median nerve, anastomoses with the ulnar nerve via a ramus communicans. Variations and overlapping areas of innervation exist; therefore, few areas of the hand can be assessed as being innervated solely by the median, ulnar, or even radial nerve.

ETIOLOGY

Inflammation of the tendon sheaths, especially in rheumatoid arthritis, represents one of the most frequent causes of nerve compression. Trauma to the hyperextended finger forces the digital nerves or their branches against the transverse metacarpal ligament. This damage may be compounded in occupations that place the fingers into hyperextension continuously. Kopell and Thompson[1] postulate that occupations using vibrating devices (saws and jackhammers) favor the development of the metacarpal tunnel syndrome. Cases involving neoplasms and digital nerve aneurysms[2] have been reported. Poulenas and Verdan[3] encouraged the use of the term "defile syndrome" rather than "tunnel syndrome" to define the compression of the digital nerves, since their anatomical investigations revealed very narrow defiles rather than tunnels.

Compression of the thumb is considered a separate entity, since the anatomy differs. Digital nerve compression of the thumb occurs most frequently in bowlers due to direct nerve compression from the bowling ball. Termed "bowler's thumb", the anatomical finding of perineural fibrosis secondary to repeated microtraumas have been reported by several investigators.[4-7]

CLINICAL SYMPTOMS AND SIGNS

Depending on whether the digitalis palmaris communis or digitalis palmaris proprius is compressed, the sensory findings will vary from sharp burning pain, hypesthesia, or paresthesias in two neighboring fingers to similar symptoms on just one side of a finger. Several fingers may be involved if more than one metacarpal tunnel is involved. Pressure between the metacarpal heads, finger hyperextension, or finger adduction may cause pain, since these aggravate the nerve compression by narrowing the tunnel.

TREATMENT

Since the predominant etiology is inflammatory in nature, treatment should be directed at reducing the perineural inflammation. Immobilization, anti-inflammatory medication, and perineural corticosteroid injections are usually successsful.[8,9] If the compression persists, some authors propose neurolysis of the affected nerves.

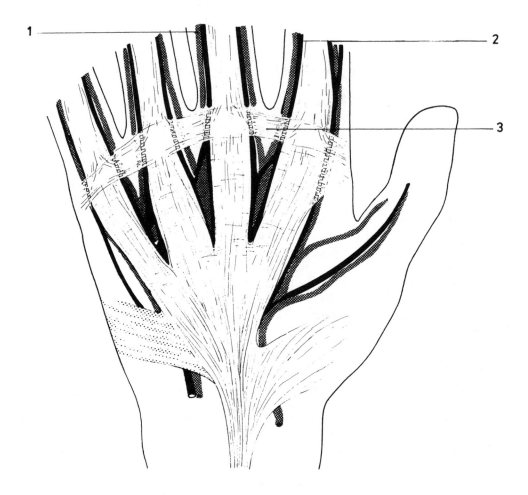

FIGURE 1.   This figure shows the arrangement of the neurovascular bundles as they leave the palm and enter the digits.
1: Proper palmar digital artery; 2: proper palmar digital nerve; 3: superficial transverse metacarpal ligament.

REFERENCES

1. Kopell, H. P. and Thompson, W. A. L., *Peripheral Entrapment Neuropathies,* William and Wilkins Co., Baltimore, 1963.
2. O'Connor, R. L., *Clin. Orthop.,* 83, 149, 1972.
3. Poulenas, I. and Verdan, C., Existe-t-il un syndrome canalaire digital?, in. *Syndromes Canalaires du Membre Supérieur,* Souquet, R., Ed., Expansion Scientifique Francaise, Paris, 1983.
4. Siegel, I. M., *JAMA,* 192, 263, 1965.
5. Marmor, L., *J. Trauma,* 6, 282, 1966.
6. Howell, A. E. and Leach, R. E., *J. Bone Joint Surg.,* 52A, 379, 1970.
7. Minkow, F. V. and Basset, F. H., *Clin. Orthop.,* 83, 115, 1972.
8. Domljan, Z., *Lijec. Vjesn.,* 91, 959, 1969.
9. Komar, J., *Alagut-szindromak,* Medicina Könyvkiado, Budapest, 1977.

Part II

TUNNEL SYNDROMES IN THE LOWER EXTREMITIES

Nerve compression in the lower extremities represent a large proportion of a physician's practice. The list of differential diagnoses can be quite long, and without appropriate testing many true diseases may be missed and many backs operated upon unnecessarily. Therefore, every patient's presenting complaint must be approached systematically. Mignoucci and Bell[1] discuss the differential diagnosis and approach to the lower back in great detail. The approach should still follow the steps outlined in the introduction. Yielding a treasure of detail, the history will indicate the avenues to search.

Lower back pain can occur simultaneously with tunnel syndromes in the lower extremity, further confusing the situation. Patients will complain of sciatica: pain radiating down from the back into the legs. The overlapping presentations of many diseases further cloud the issue. Degenerative or traumatic disc disease, spinal stenosis, referred pain from bony disease in this extended region, peripheral vascular disease, malingering, psychiatric disturbances, trauma, infection, inflammation, tumors (intrinsic or extrinsic to the nerve), neuropathies, or hormonal and metabolic disturbances, can masquerade as peripheral nerve entrapment. Saal et al.[2] suggested that nerve irritation leads to substance release into the spinal cord, increasing the sensitivity of nearby nerves to pain.

Initial treatment of lower back pain involves bed rest, anti-inflammatories, analgesics, physical therapy, modalities, education, and job modification. Typically, 50% of patients with lower back pain recover within a month.[3] In fact, less than 3 to 10% of all patients with unrelenting sciatica ever require surgical intervention.[4] Evaluation of patients with chronic back pain does not typically yield a surgically correctable lesion;[4] therefore, cautious intervention is required. However, these same patients become quite familiar with physicians' expectations and can present quite intriguing symptoms. From among all these patients comes the select group with tunnel syndromes of the lower extremity.

REFERENCES

1. Mignoucci, L. and Bell, G., *The Spine,* W. B. Saunders, Philadelphia, 1991.
2. Saal, J. A., Dillingham, M. F., Gamburd, R. S., and Fanton, G. S., *Spine,* 13, 926, 1985.
3. Andersson, G. J. B., Svensson, H. O., and Oden, A., *Spine,* 8, 880, 1983.
4. Frymoyer, J. W., *N. Engl. J. Med.,* 318(5), 291-300, 1988.

LUMBOSACRAL TUNNEL SYNDROME

Compression of the fifth lumbar nerve root represents one of the most common complaints of patients with lower back pain and sciatica. While this nerve root is commonly involved by a herniated disc or spinal stenosis, the fifth nerve root can be compressed after it leaves the intervertebral foramen and crosses the alla of the ilium under the iliolumbar ligament (Figure 1). This region is commonly known as the lumbosacral tunnel.

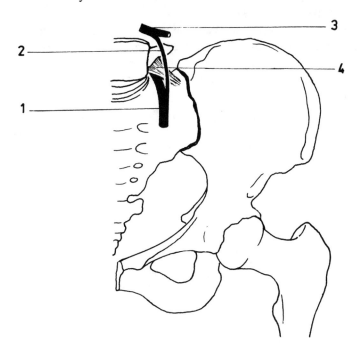

FIGURE 1.   This figure gives the anatomical relationships of the lumbosacral tunnel.
1: L5 root; 2: communicating branch of the sympathetic trunk; 3: L4 root; 4: lumbosacral ligament.

ANATOMY

Its large fibrous band forming the medial side of the fibro-osseus tunnel, the iliolumbar ligament originates from the fifth lumbar vertebra and inserts on the upper border and anterior surface of the alla. Nathan et al.[1] state that the ligament develops in everyone but varies in its width, thickness, and shape. The ligament's origin may be both the body of L5 and its transverse process (73%), the body solely (20%), or the transverse process solely (7%). The alla or the wing of the ilium forms the posterior wall of the fibro-osseus tunnel.

The fifth lumbar nerve leaves the intervertebral foramen and runs inferolaterally, crossing the upper border of the ilium before reaching the anterior surface of the sacrum. Over this course, the nerve courses under the iliolumbar ligament. Sympathetic nerve branches pierce the superior border of the ligament and join with the nerve. The fourth lumbar nerve root runs over the anterior surface of the iliolumbar ligament to join the fifth nerve root as it exits from the inferior border of the ligament. The lumbosacral tunnel also contains branches of the iliolumbar arteries and veins and may even contain a venous plexus. Lumbosacral nerve-root anomalies are not rare in this region.[2]

ETIOLOGY

As in all tunnel syndromes, nerve compression occurs when disease processes alter the volume of the lumbosacral tunnel. Marginal osteophytes on L5 and S1 can be so exuberant that they can form a compressive anteromedial wall.[3,4] Thickening of the ligament can flatten the nerve against the posterior ilium wall.[1] Intrinsic and extrinsic neural tumors will decrease the space in the tunnel. Additionally, disorders of the tunnel's vascular components may compress the nerve. These include aneurysms, tortuosities, and venous dilatations.[1] Regional inflammation can lead to local tissue edema and compression. Bony changes including primary and secondary tumors of the ilium and spine, fractures of the pelvic ring and sacrum, and motion of the sacroiliac and lumbosacral spine may produce symptomatic nerve compression.[5]

CLINICAL SYMPTOMS AND SIGNS

The symptoms and signs of lumbosacral tunnel syndrome are found in the L5 distribution. One will find decreased sensation and pain in the L5 dermatome. Weakness and atrophy usually is unobserved. Therefore, the diagnosis of the lumbosacral tunnel syndrome requires exclusion of the other causes of L5 radiculopathy, as mentioned earlier.

TREATMENT

Conservative therapy should be applied along the accepted courses for relief of radicular pain.[6] Chayen et al.[7] describe the use of anesthetic blocks. Surgical release remains the last resort, with care being taken not to include the fourth lumbar nerve while sectioning the iliolumbar ligament.

REFERENCES

1. Nathan, H., Weizenbluth, M., and Halperin, N., *Int. Orthop.*, 6, 197, 1982.
2. Postacchini, F., Urso, S., and Ferro, L., *J. Bone Joint Surg.*, 64A, 721, 1982.
3. Danforth, M. S. and Wilson, P. P., *J. Bone Joint Surg.*, 7, 109, 1925.
4. Epstein, J. A. and Epstein, B. S., *Bull. N.Y. Acad. Med.*, 35, 370, 1959.
5. Mitchell, G. A. G., *J. Bone Joint Surg.*, 16, 233, 1934.
6. Epstein, J. A., *J. Neurosurg.*, 17, 991, 1960.
7. Chayen, D., Nathan, H., and Chayen, M., *Anesthesia,* 45, 95, 1976.

ILIACUS MUSCLE SYNDROME
(SYNDROME OF THE FEMORAL NERVE
IN THE MUSCULARIS LACUNA)

The femoral neurovascular bundle and the iliopsoas muscle pass under the inguinal ligament to supply the leg. The iliac fascia forms an iliopectineal arch that connects the inguinal ligament to the iliopubic or iliopectineal eminence and divides the space beneath the inguinal ligament (Figure 1). The lacuna vasorum or vascular tunnel lies medial to the arch. Through the lateral space of the lacuna muscularis runs the femoral nerve and the iliopsoas muscles. Relatively rigid, the lacuna muscularis represents a tunnel whose walls are the iliac bone, the iliopsoas muscle, the iliopectineal arch, and the inguinal ligament. Described by Aichroth and Rowe-Jones in 1971,[1] the syndrome of the iliacus muscle, or the iliacus tunnel syndrome, occurs with femoral nerve compression.

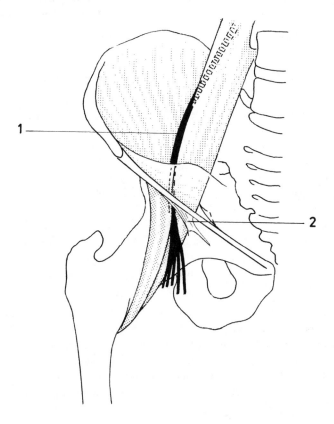

FIGURE 1.   This figure shows the course of the femoral nerve (1) as it crosses the iliacus muscle and pelvis to pass near the iliopectineal arch (2), to supply the leg.

ANATOMY

The femoral nerve originates from roots L2, L3, and L4 below the psoas muscle. Passing between the iliacus and psoas muscles, the nerve supplies both muscles and enters the leg with the combined iliopsoas tendon under the inguinal ligament. One of two terminal divisions of the

TABLE 1
Proposed Etiologies for Femoral Nerve Compression

Etiology	Author
Extrinsic Hysterectomy	Gumpertz, 1896[3] Adler et al., 1956[4] Krone, 1972[5] Komar, 1973[2] Kvist-Poulsen and Borel, 1982[6]
Retractor placement	Buchbender and Weiss, 1961[7]
Spontaneous retroperitoneal bleed	Seddon, 1930[8] Tellroth, 1939[9] Hall, 1961[10] Lang, 1966[11] Fearn, 1968[12] Cianci and Piscattelli, 1969[13] Mastroianni and Roberts, 1983[14]
Iliacus or psoas muscles bleed	Goodfellow et al., 1967[15] Uncini et al., 1981[16]
Intrinsic (hematoma within the nerve)	Bigelow and Graves, 1952[17]
Functional (in sport or action) Hip hyperextension	Aichroth and Rowe-Jones, 1971[1] Koll, 1957[18] Luft, 1963[19]

femoral nerve, the superficial nerve branch supplies motor rami to the pectineus and sartorius muscles as well as sensation to the anterior thigh via the anterior cutaneous ramus. The deep branch supplies the quadriceps femoris musculature and produces the saphenous nerve, which supplies sensation to the medial thigh, leg, and foot. All anterior thigh muscles except the tensor fascia lata are innervated by the femoral nerve. Sensory disturbances due to femoral nerve compromise would be seen over the anterior thigh, the anterior medial area of the knee, the medial leg, and the medial portion of the foot.

ETIOLOGY

Since the femoral nerve lies in the pelvic basin, surgical procedures within the pelvis are the most common cause of femoral nerve compression. Hematomas and dynamic relationships can also compress the nerve. Bleeding within the nerve sheath produces intrinsic compression, whereas bleeding external to the sheath can still narrow the tunnel significantly (see Table 1).

One may postulate that arteriovenous malformations, vascular aneurysms, muscle tumors, bony disruptions due to traums, or hernias can also lead to femoral nerve compromise.

CLINICAL SYMPTOMS AND SIGNS

Symptoms can be predicted using one's knowledge of the femoral nerve's anatomy and the level of compressive lesion. Patients with high lesions (often termed paresis of the superior type) have difficulty standing from a seated position due to iliopsoas muscle weakness. High lesions will also compromise lower femoral nerve function. Patients with iliacus tunnel syndrome (paresis of the inferior type) have difficulty extending their knee. They also have hypotrophy of the anterior thigh compartment. Hip extension aggravates the pain, while other movements of the hip are painless. The patellar reflex typically disappears. Sensory disturbances will be appreciated throughout the femoral nerve's dermatome. Radiculopathy would present segmental sensory disturbances. Quadripes hypotrophy has neither the sensory disturbances nor the pain associated with iliacus tunnel syndrome.

TREATMENT

Komar[2] recommends conservative therapy, since the risks of surgical exploration outweighed its benefits. Physical therapy may stabilize the quadriceps hypotrophy. The best treatment lies in avoidance of surgical damage during pelvic procedures and reversal of coagulopathies and other causes.

REFERENCES

1. Aichroth, P. and Rowe-Jones, D. C., *Br. J. Surg.,* 58, 833, 1971.
2. Komar, J., *Alagut-szindromak,* Medicina Könyvkiado, Budapest, 1977.
3. Gumpertz, K., *Dtsch. Med. Wochenschr.,* 22, 504, 1896.
4. Adler, E., Jarus, A., and Magora, A., *Acta Psych. Neurol. Scand.,* 31, 1, 1956.
5. Krone, H. A., *Zentralbl. Gynakol.,* 94, 697, 1972.
6. Kvist-Poulsen, H. and Borel, J., *Obstet. Gynecol.,* 60, 516, 1982.
7. Buchbender, E. and Weiss, R., *Nervenarzt,* 32, 413, 1961.
8. Seddon, S., *Brain,* 53, 306, 1930.
9. Tellroth, A., *Acta Chir. Scand.,* 82, 1, 1939.
10. Hall, M., *Br. J. Haematol.,* 7, 340, 1961.
11. Lang, L. S., *Br. Med. J.,* 2, 93, 1966.
12. Fearn, C. B., *Br. Med. J.,* 4, 97, 1968.
13. Cianci, P. E. and Piscatelli, R. L., *JAMA,* 210, 1100, 1969.
14. Mastroianni, P. P. and Roberts, M. P., *Neurosurgery,* 13, 44, 1983.
15. Goodfellow, J., Fearn, C. B., and Mathes, J. M., *J. Bone Joint Surg.,* 49B, 748, 1967.
16. Uncini, A., Tonali, P., Falappa, P., and Danza, F. M., *J. Neurol.,* 266, 137, 1981.
17. Bigelow, N. H. and Graves, R. W., *Arch. Neurol. Psychiatr.,* 68, 819, 1952.
18. Koll, J. F., *Nervenzart,* 28, 30, 1957.
19. Luft, H., *Nervenarzt,* 34, 457, 1963.

OBTURATOR TUNNEL SYNDROME

While leaving the pelvis and entering the thigh, the obturator nerve passes through a fibro-osseus tunnel, the obturator tunnel. Compression of the obturator nerve can mimic many different disorders, ranging from herniated discs to nerve compression at other levels in the pelvis.

ANATOMY

Originating from the second, third, and fourth lumbar nerve roots of the lumbar plexus, the obturator nerve passes below the psoas muscle, crosses over the sacroiliac joint, and runs along the pelvic wall to reach the obturator tunnel (Figure 1).

The obturator sulcus of the pubic bone forms the roof of the tunnel, with the floor consisting of the internal and external obturator muscles. The obturator membrane separates the muscles and joins with their fascias to create an inelastic floor of the oblique tunnel. The obturator artery, two veins, and multiple lymph nodes can be found alongside the obturator nerve in the tunnel. Within the tunnel, the nerve divides into an anterior or superficial branch, a posterior or deep branch, and a branch to the external obturator muscle.

As the nerve exits the tunnel, the anterior and the posterior branches are separated by the adductor brevis muscle. The anterior branch innervates the pectineus, adductor longus, adductor brevis, and gracillis muscles. Its terminal branch supplies sensory fibers to the skin of the medial thigh. The posterior branch supplies the adductor brevis and the adductor magnus muscles. The obturator nerve also supplies sensation to the knee joint and the medial side of the knee. Lolić-Draganić and Ilić[1] estimate that 9% of individuals have an accessory obturator nerve that leaves the pubis through either muscular or vascular passages (lacunae musculorum or vasorum, Figure 2).

ETIOLOGY

The course of the obturator nerve places it at risk from disorders of all organ systems in the pelvis as well as from compression within the tunnel. The nerve may be compressed within the true pelvis by pelvic fractures, pelvic hematomas secondary to anticoagulation or trauma,[2] retroperitoneal masses,[3] and intrapelvic tumors. Normal life events like pregnancy can develop complications that lead to obturator nerve or obstetrical palsy.[4,5]

While the obturator tunnel is well protected from direct trauma by neighboring muscles, neuropathy due to direct damage may occur. Complications of genitourological surgery or total hip arthroplasty[6,7] may traumatize the nerve in its tunnel. Anticoagulation may also lead to minor bleeds within the tunnel[2] which still leads to compression, since the tunnel size requires that any increase in size by any component necessitates a decrease in the other components. Of all the tunnel components, the obturator nerve is the least tolerant of compression. Obturator hernias or tissue edema due to inflammation can also lead to nerve compression. Kopell and Thompson[8] describe obturator tunnel syndrome related to inflammatory changes of the pubic bone in osteitis pubis.

CLINICAL SYMPTOMS AND SIGNS

While osteitis pubis causes mild local pain, obturator tunnel syndrome causes strong nonlocalized pain and resting pain with radiation from the symphysis pubis to the knee. Medial knee pain, known as Howship Romberg's symptom[9] develops with nerve compression. Occasionally sharp pain may be felt in the posteromedial knee. This area receives innervation from the posterior obturator nerve branch. With prolonged compression, adductor paresis may develop. However, the adductor longus muscle and the adductor magnus muscle receive partial

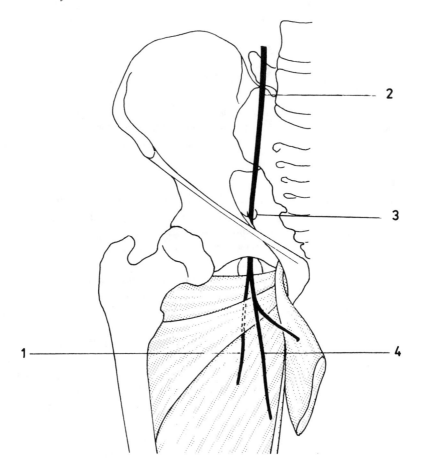

FIGURE 1.   This figure illustrates the relationship of the obturator nerve and its branches to the internal rotators of the hip and the adductor muscles.
1: Posterior (profundus) branch of the obturator nerve; 2: obturator nerve; 3: obturator canal; 4: anterior (superficial) branch of the obturator nerve.

innervation from the femoral nerve and the sciatic nerve, respectively. Adductor paresis produces a characteristic gait where circumduction of the affected leg occurs. Deep nonlocalized pain and spasm may develop among the adductor muscles. Some investigators question whether adductor spasm can lead to obturator tunnel syndrome.

In review, medial knee pain[3] or adductor spasm combined with medial thigh and knee pain[10] can be considered characteristic for obturator tunnel syndrome.

TREATMENT

Primary obturator tunnel syndrome can be treated conservatively with physical therapy and rest. However, obturator tunnel syndrome secondary to pelvic pathology requires treatment of the cause. With the exception of coagulopathies, these causes must be treated surgically via a pelvic approach.

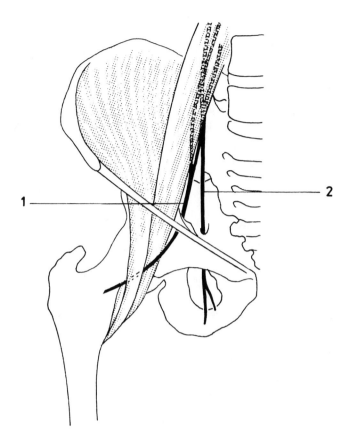

FIGURE 2.   Variations in the obturator nerve can occur with an accessory obturator nerve (1) crossing the pelvis in a separate location from the obturator nerve (2).

REFERENCES

1. Lolić-Draganić, V. and Ilić, A., *Acta Orthop. Lugosl.*, 3, 361, 1972.
2. Susens, G. P., Hendrickson, C. G., Mulder, M. J., and Sams, B., *Ann. Intern. Med.*, 59, 575, 1968.
3. Misoul, C., Nerve Injuries and entrapment syndromes of the lower extremity, in *Principles of Orthopaedic Practice*, Dee, R., Ed., McGraw-Hill, New York, 1989.
4. Oppenheim, H., *Lehrbuch der Nervenkrankheiten*, S. Kagerer, Berlin, 1923.
5. Clark, J. M. P., *J. Bone Joint Surg.*, 47B, 806, 1965.
6. Weber, E. R., Daube, J. R., and Coventry, M. B., *J. Bone Joint Surg.*, 58A, 66, 1976.
7. Siliski, J. M. and Scott, R. D., *J. Bone Joint Surg.*, 67A, 1225, 1985.
8. Kopell, H. P. and Thompson, W. A. L., *N. Engl. J. Med.*, 262, 56, 1960.
9. Komar, J., *Alagut-szindromak*, Medicina Könyvkiado, Budapest, 1977.
10. Lam, S. J. S., *Guy's Hosp. Rep.*, 117, 49, 1968.

PIRIFORMIS MUSCLE SYNDROME

The sciatic nerve passes through the greater sciatic foramen in close proximity to the piriformis muscle (Figure 1). Compression in this fibro-osseus tunnel may result in the clinical picture of the piriformis syndrome. In 1928, Yeoman described the importance of the neuromuscular relationship in the development of lumbosacral neuralgias.[1] Since the L4,5 and S1,2 distributions are affected, the list of differential diagnoses can be quite broad.

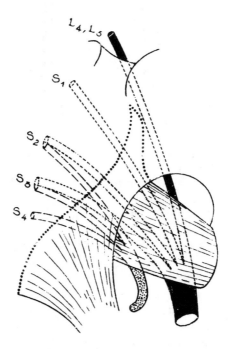

FIGURE 1.   As shown above, the sciatic nerve lies in close proximity to the piriformis muscle and can even run through it in several variations.

ANATOMY

The sacrospinal and the sacrotuberous ligaments connect the ischial spine and the ischial tuberosity, respectively, to the sacrum and delineate two foramens: the greater (foramen ischiadicum majus) and the lesser (foramen ischiadiacum minus) sciatic foramens. The greater (incisura ischiadica major) and the lesser (incisura ischiadica minor) sciatic notches lie at the apex of each foramen along the posterior ischial border. The majority of important structures connecting the gluteal region with the pelvis run throught the greater sciatic foramen; therefore, this area has been known as the hilus of the gluteus or the Gibraltar of the gluteus. The piriformis muscle splits the foramen into the suprapiriformis region and the infrapiriformis region. The superior gluteal nerve and vessels leave through the suprapiriformis region.

The infrapiriformis region or foramen is triangular in shape, delineated by the inferior margin of the piriformis muscle superiorly, the sacrospinous ligament inferiorly, and the bony margin of the greater sciatic notch laterally. Two groups of neurovascular structures leave the

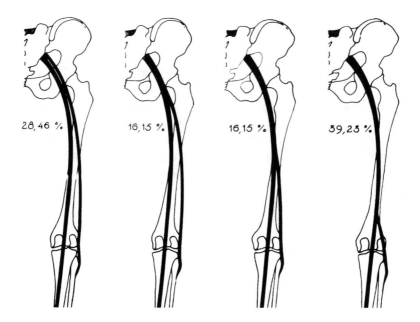

FIGURE 2.   These four illustrations reveal the most common variations in the form taken by the sciatic nerve as it courses down the lower extremity. The most common forms occur with the sciatic nerve dividing before leaving the pelvis or just proximal to the knee.

pelvis through this region. The medial group includes the pudendal neurovascular bundle. The lateral group consists of the sciatic nerve, the inferior gluteal nerve, the posterior cutaneous nerve of the thigh, and the inferior gluteal vessels. The sciatic nerve represents two terminal nerves of the sacral plexus: the tibial nerve, which is the ventral portion of the plexus (L4,5;S1,2), and the common peroneal nerve, which is the dorsal portion of the sacral plexus (L4,5;S1,2). While considered an extremely important nerve, the sciatic nerve enters the thigh as one or two nerves. Studies by Pećina[2] revealed intrapelvic division in 26.5% of the cases, postforamen division in 4.6% of the cases, division at the inferior border of the gluteus maximus muscle in 11.5% of the cases, and division in the thigh in the rest of the cases (Figure 2). Occasionally, the common peroneal nerve may pass through the piriformis muscle (long, flat, or pear like) separating the muscle into two bellies.[3-9] The piriformis muscle has been shown to exist in two bellies in 18% of the population.[2] The sacral plexus and branches of the internal iliac artery lie between the rectum and the piriformis muscle, which covers the anterior surface of the sacrum.

Surgical approaches in the gluteal region, especially with hip surgery, use the piriformis muscle for orientation, since it connects the sacrum and the greater trochanter of the femur. The position and direction of the upper muscular margin can be found by following the superior iliotrochanteric line, which connects the posterior superior iliac spine with the apex of the greater trochanter (Figure 3). The inferior iliotrochanteric line runs parallel and 3 cm distal to the superior iliotrochanteric line. The inferior line will indicate the upper margin of the infra-piriformis foramen or region.

The contents of the foramen and their relative volumes play a major role in the development of nerve compression. The size of the piriformis muscle belly may vary greatly, thereby narrowing the foramen. In up to 50% of the population, a synovial bursa may exist between the tendon of the piriformis muscle and the bone. The piriformis muscle functions to externally rotate the hip as well as to help extend the hip. With the hip already flexed, the piriformis muscle acts as a hip abductor. If the thigh is fixed, the muscle acts to rotate the pelvis to the activated side and backwards. The common peroneal nerve can pass through the piriformis muscle in 21%

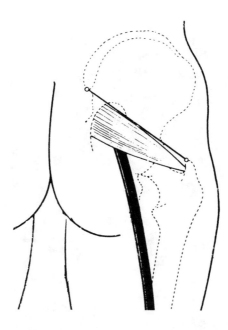

FIGURE 3.   This figure indicates the projection
of the piriformis muscle on the surface anatomy of
the gluteal region.

of the population (Figure 4); however only in 5% of these people does the muscle actually divide
to allow the nerve to pass (Figures 5 and 6). The divided muscle actually plays an important role
in the development of the piriformis syndrome.

ETIOLOGY

Multiple etiologies have been proposed to explain the compression or irritation of the sciatic
nerve as it courses distally. While all have been proposed as etiologies, basic anatomical
relationships, direct and indirect trauma, inflammation, and local ischemia probably combine
to induce the piriformis muscle syndrome.

Yeoman [1] emphasized the anatomical relationship of the sciatic nerve and the piriformis
muscle. The development of the syndrome secondary to muscle irritation can be divided into the
four groups, shown in Table 1. Many authors have discussed the relationship of sacroiliac joint
disease and the lumbosacral plexus leading to ischialgia;[10,11] however, Yeoman [1] was the first to
link sacroiliac disease with piriformis muscle spasm. Freiberg and Vinke[12] and others have since
seconded this opinion.[6,12a,13] Levin[14] described the anatomical position of the piriformis muscle
during the Lasegue-Lazarevic test. At approximately 20°, the muscle is stretched and compression may occur. In some patients with a clinical picture of lumboischialgia of unknown etiology,
the test becomes positive at small angles where only the muscle, not the nerve, is stretched. Static
disorders of the lumbosacral spine and hip can produce symptoms.[15] Flexion contracture at the
hip may produce lumbar lordosis. Increased tension of the pelvifemoral muscles develops as the
muscles try to stabilize the pelvis and spine in the new position. The involved muscles
hypertrophy to handle the tension; however, the bony foramens do not enlarge. This leads to a
decrease in available space for the neurovascular structures With neural tissue being the least
tolerant to compression of the neurovascular bundle, neurological signs develop earlier than
vascular signs. The infrapiriformis foramen narrows with piriformis hypertrophy and may lead
to sciatic nerve compression.[2,16,17] If the sciatic nerve passes between the two tendinous heads
of the piriformis, compression occurs with muscle stretch during internal hip rotation rather than
muscle contraction (Figures 4).

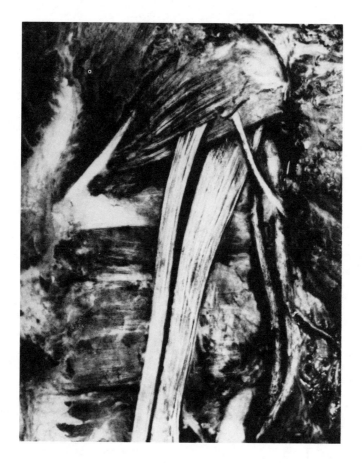

FIGURE 4.   This photograph reveals one of the variations in the form of the sciatic nerve. This specimen shows the common peroneal nerve passing through the piriformis muscle.

TABLE 1
Postulated Etiologies for the Development of the Piriformis Muscle Syndrome Due to the Irritation of the Nerve

1. Muscle spasm secondary to irritation of the piriformis at either its origin by sacroiliac disease or at its insertion by bursitis or trochanteric diseases

2. Inflammatory or degenerative changes of the muscle, tendon, or fascia

3. Degeneration or deformities affecting the bony origin or insertion of the muscle

4. Anomalies in the nerve's course through the muscle or between the muscle's tendon and the bone (the vascular structures may also be affected)

Trauma, either direct or indirect, can lead to compression of the piriformis muscle by scarring, spasm, or simply the muscle mass of the gluteus maximus muscle. Robinson[18] and Pace and Nagle[19] postulated that trauma in the sacroiliac or gluteal region can lead to piriformis

TABLE 2
Several Etiologies of the Piriformis Syndrome

Author	Etiology
Yeoman, 1928[1]	Piriformis muscle spasm secondary to sacro-iliac disease
Robinson, 1947[18]	Trauma in the sacroiliac or gluteal region
Steinbracher	Trauma, fibrous adhesions
Hoff, 1949[30]	Inflammation of the synovial bursa
Topličanec and Dürrigl, 1966[31]	Inflammation of the synovial bursa
Kopell and Thompson, 1960[15]	Passage of the common peroneal nerve through the muscle belly
Pećina, 1969[2]	Vascular compromise due to direct compression
Pećina, 1969, 1975, 1979[2,16,17]	Anatomical relationships of the muscle and sciatic nerve: compression due to discordance between the size of the sciatic foramen and the muscle, position of the nerve under the tendon and above the bone, or between the two heads of the divided piriformis muscle

syndrome. Steiner et al.[13] felt that adhesions between the neural and the muscular fibrous sheaths would lead to compression when the now combined unit distorts with muscular contraction.

Inflammation can lead to changes in the relationships between all the structures in this area. As shown in Table 2, many authors have discussed the possibility of muscular spasm with changes in the synovial bursa. Inflammation of any structure in a narrow area can lead to compression or scarring, which will lead to distortion with motion.

Besides the direct compression of the nerve, compression of the vessels supplying the nerve may lead to the piriformis syndrome.[2] A branch of the inferior gluteal artery, a. commitans n. ischiadici, and the corresponding veins join the nerve as it crosses the inferior margin of the piriformis. Constant or repeated muscle spasm can compress the vessels and lead to vascular congestion or ischemia in the sheath. These changes can produce pain along the nerve.

CLINICAL SYMPTOMS AND SIGNS

The piriformis syndrome has many similarities with and overlaps with symptoms of lower back pain, ischialgias, vascular disease, and lower extremity pathologies. Pain and paresthesias can present along the entire sciatic nerve. In time, burning sensations, hypesthesia, or anesthesia may develop. Motor weakness or hypotrophy may be included in the presentation. If the sympathetic branches are compressed, trophic changes in the skin will be appreciated. Frequently, diagnosis requires eliminating other causes of sciatic nerve impingement or irritation based on the historical and physical findings described in Table 3.

Pain in the sacral or gluteal region remains the most constant symptom. The pain increases with sitting or walking and decreases with lying supine. However, not all authors concur. Lam[20] stressed that lumbosacral pressure is not present but that nerve irritability in the gluteal region exists. Robinson[18] described the pain and irritability as originating in the sacroiliac joint and the region of the greater sciatic foramen and the piriformis. Infiltration of the muscle with anesthetic may alleviate the pain and eliminate the symptoms by relieving muscle spasm. Rectal examination with palpation of the piriformis provides an objective evaluation of the muscle's

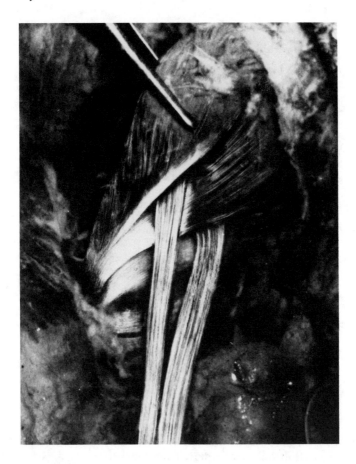

FIGURE 5.   This photograph reveals a second variation in the form taken by the common peroneal nerve as it courses between the tendinous portions of the piriformis muscle.

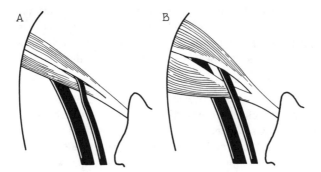

FIGURE 6.   Dynamic or functional anatomy has been postulated as a cause of the piriformis syndrome. This figure illustrates the change in the piriformis muscle when stretched passively or contracted actively. (A) In passive stretching of the divided piriformis muscle by internal thigh rotation, the tendinous portions compress the nerve; (B) in active contraction of the muscle in external rotation, the space between the tendons enlarges and the nerve is free to pass. These changes must be noted, since these relationships depend on the actual course taken by the nerve.

TABLE 3
Several Differentiating Symptoms and Signs of the Piriformis Syndrome

- No pain in the lumbosacral region
- Peripheral nerve distribution irritation, not radicular in origin
- Irritability on palpation of the greater sciatic foramen (region between the greater trochanter and the posterior superior iliac spine)
- Palpable mass (or swelling) over the region of the piriformis muscle with exacerbation of pain
- Piriformis muscle spasm appreciated by rectal exam
- Positive Lasegue-Lazarevic sign at 25°
- Increased pain with internal rotation of the hip or hip flexion with an extended knee
- Decreased pain with external rotation of the hip

spasm.[21,22] Additionally, a rectal examination allows a quick screening for rectal and lower pelvic pathology. Pelvic and lower back disease may require further studies, including laboratory and radiographic evaluations. Karl et al.[23] describe the scintigraphic appearance of the syndrome in one patient.

Several physical examination maneuvers elicit symptoms. The Gowers-Bonnet test seeks to elicit pain with hip flexion, knee flexion, and internal rotation. While not pathognomonic, this test seeks to stretch the piriformis. A modification of this test, as described by Pećina[16] and Komar,[24] has the patient bend forward while standing with knees extended to passively stretch the piriformis and the sciatic nerve.

TREATMENT

Conservative therapy consisting of physiotherapy, corticosteroid and anesthetic injections, and anti-inflammatory medication may be tried to alleviate muscle spasm.[18,19,25-28] Corticosteroid and anesthetic injections into the synovial bursa under the piriformis at its insertion into the greater trochanter may be repeated to bring relief. Therefore, injection can be considered both diagnostic and therapeutic. Treatment of sacroileitis, if present, will bring relief. Surgical therapy must be initiated within 6 to 8 months of presentation. If the compression is due to muscle position or stretch or size, sectioning of the piriformis muscle tendon near its insertion will release the nerve.[29] Loss of piriformis action does not cause any noticeable functional disturbance and in most patients will lead to disappearance of symptoms.

REFERENCES

1. Yeoman, W., *Lancet,* 2, 1119, 1928.
2. Pećina, M., *Oštećenja zivćanog stabla i ogranaka ishijadikusa uvjetovana posebnim topografskoanatomskim odnosima,* disertacija, Medicinski Fafultet, Zagreb, 1969.
3. Mouret, J., *Montepell. Méd.,* 2, 230, 1893.
4. Vallois, H. V., *C. R. Assoc. Anat.,* 24, 519, 1929.
5. Berkol, N., Mouchet, A., and Gögen, H., *Annis Anat. Pathol.,* 12, 596, 1935.
6. Beaton, L. E. and Anson, B. J., *J. Bone Joint Surg.,* 20, 686, 1938.
7. Lazorthes, G., *Le Systéme Nerveux Périphérique,* Masson, Paris, 1955.
8. Odajima, G. and Kurihara, T., *Excerpta Med.,* 17, 9, 1963.
9. Ilić, A., Mrvaljević, D., Blasotić, M., Dordević Camba, V., and Marintkovic, S., *Acta Orthop. Lugosl.,* 7, 163, 1976.
10. Danforth, M. S. and Wilson, P. D., *J. Bone Joint Surg.,* 23, 109, 1925.
11. Hershey, C. D., *JAMA,* 122, 983, 1943.
12. Freiberg, A. H. and Vinke, T. H., *J. Bone Joint Surg.,* 16, 126, 1934.

12a. Freiberg, A. H., *Arch. Surg.,* 34, 337, 1937.
13. Steiner, C., Staubs, C., Gagon, M., and Buhlinger, C., *J. Am. Osteopath. Assoc.,* 87, 318, 1987.
14. Levin, Ph., *JAMA,* 82, 965, 1924.
15. Kopell, H. P. and Thompson, W. A. L., *N. Engl. J. Med.,* 262, 56, 1960.
16. Pećina, M., *Acta Orthop. Lugosl.,* 6, 196, 1975.
17. Pećina, M., *Acta Anat. (Basel),* 105, 181, 1979.
18. Robinson, D. R., *Am. J. Surg.,* 73, 355, 1947.
19. Pace, J. B. and Nagle, D., *West J. Med.,* 124, 435, 1979.
20. Lam, S. J. S., *Guy's Hosp. Rep.,* 117, 449, 1968.
21. Synek, V. M., *Clin. Exp. Neurol.,* 23, 31, 1987.
22. Pfeifer, Th. and Fitz, W. F. K., *Z. Orthop.,* 127, 691, 1989.
23. Karl, R. D. Jr, et al., *Clin. Nucl. Med.,* 10, 361, 1985.
24. Komar, J., *Alagut-szindromak,* Medicina Könyvkiado, Budapest, 1977.
25. Haggart, G. E., *J. Bone Joint Surg.,* 20, 851 1938.
26. Wynat, G. M., *Can. Anaesth. Soc. J.,* 26, 305, 1979.
27. Noftal, F., *Can. J. Surg.,* 31, 210, 1988.
28. Misoul, C., Nerve injuries and entrapment syndromes of the lower extremity, in *Principles of Orthopaedic Practice, Dee,* R., Ed., McGraw-Hill, New York, 1989.
29. Solheim, L. F., Siewers, P., and Paus, B., *Acta Orthop. Scand.,* 52, 73, 1981.
30. Hoff, H., *Wien Med. Wochenschr.,* 99, 455, 1949.
31. Topličanec, M. and Dürrigl, Th., *Lijec. Vjesn.,* 88, 167, 1966.

MERALGIA PARESTHETICA
(SYNDROME OF THE INGUINAL LIGAMENT;
SYNDROME OF THE LATERAL FEMORAL CUTANEOUS NERVE)

The lateral femoral cutaneous nerve passes through two fibrous tunnel consisting of the inguinal ligament and the fascia lata to reach the anterolateral thigh. Described initially as Roth's meralgy[1] and Bernhard's syndrome,[2,3] meralgia paresthetica occurs with nerve compression in the fibrous tunnels or nerve stretching. Mumenthaler and Schliack[4] used its anatomical location to categorize the syndrome of the inguinal ligament.

ANATOMY

Solely a sensory nerve, the lateral femoral cutaneous nerve originates from the L2 and L3 nerve roots, passes under the psoas muscle, and emerges laterally to cross the ilium buried in a fibrous tunnel formed by a doubling in the iliacus muscle's fascia. As shown in Figure 1, the nerve courses towards the medial aspect of the anterior superior iliac spine and bends through the inguinal ligament at an angle of 70 to 90°. At this point, the nerve divides into a thick anterior and thin posterior branch. Leaving the pelvis in this fashion, the anterior branch pierces the fascia lata to innervate the skin of the lateral thigh (Figure 2). The posterior branch runs deep under the tensor fascia lata muscle to innervate the skin of the gluteal region.

Stevens[5] and Ghent[6,7] describe the following four variations of the lateral femoral cutaneous nerve: first, the nerve passes under the inguinal ligament; second, the nerve makes a sharp turn when crossing the iliac fascia; third, the nerve passes through the sartorius muscle; and fourth, the nerve courses laterally and behind the anterior superior iliac spine.

ETIOLOGY

Vulnerable to compression and stretching from its origin under the psoas muscle until it exits through the inguinal ligament and the fascia lata, the lateral femoral cutaneous nerve can be damaged by multiple etiologies including tumor, trauma, and surgical complications, as shown in Table 1. Compression above the fascial tunnels and in the tunnels can be considered upper and lower forms of the syndrome.[8]

To explain meralgia paresthetica without any identifiable cause, Kopell and Thompson[9] postulate that the nerve can be damaged by acute or chronic stretching. Since the lateral femoral cutaneous nerve is fixed both at its origin and at the fascial tunnels, leg length changes, scoliosis, increased tension of the abdominal musculature and facia lata (due to long periods of standing), trunk or leg hyperextension, and surgery may damage the nerve. In cadaver studies, Nathan[10] found that approximately 50% of all lateral femoral cutaneous nerves were thickened where they had pierced the inguinal ligament.

CLINICAL SYMPTOMS AND SIGNS

Characteristic symptoms consist of paresthesia, burning pain, and dysthesias aggravated by even the touch of clothing or leg extension while sleeping. Patients even avoid placing keys or objects over the affected thigh.[11] Some investigators encourage the limitation of meralgia paresthetica's definition to sensory complaints, not the signs.[8] Clinical examination will reveal hypesthesia, trophic skin changes with long-standing compression, hair loss, and a positive inversed Lasegue's sign. Seeking to elicit pain over the thigh, the inversed Lasegue's sign is performed by flexing the knee and extending the hip with the patient in a lateral position (similar to Menel's procedure). Local pressure over the inguinal ligament, especially close to the anterior superior iliac spine in the lower form of this syndrome, may produce pain or local

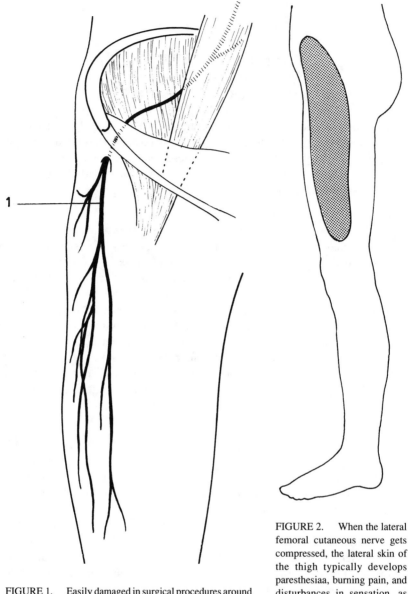

1

FIGURE 1.   Easily damaged in surgical procedures around the hip, the lateral femoral cutaneous nerve (1) passes anteriorly to the anterior superior iliac spine before coursing laterally over the thigh.

FIGURE 2.   When the lateral femoral cutaneous nerve gets compressed, the lateral skin of the thigh typically develops paresthesiaa, burning pain, and disturbances in sensation, as shown above. Some patients will not keep anything in their pockets on the affected side.

irritation in the nerve's distribution, similar to a Tinel's sign. Evaluated in patients using their unaffected leg as a control, electromyographic studies effectively show nerve compression on the affected side.[12] The differential diagnosis should include intraspinal or extraspinal radiculopathies of the L2 and L3 nerve roots and lumbar plexus pathology.[13,14] Etiologies causing the upper form of the syndrome may be hard to identify without a computed tomography (CT) or magnetic resonance imaging (MRI) of the abdomen and pelvis. Thermography is also useful in helping diagnose meralgia paresthetica.[15]

TREATMENT

Treatment must address the underlying compression. Compression in the upper form requires decompression. The lower form, affecting the fascial tunnels, requires relief of tension

TABLE 1
Proposed Etiologies of Meralgia Paresthetica and Their Investigators

Etiology	Investigators
Retroperitoneal hematoma or tumor	Flowers, 1968[17]
Iliopsoas muscle abscess	
Abdominal aortic aneurysm	Carayon and Gruet, 1969[18]
Abdominal/inguinal surgery	Moscona and Hirshowitz, 1980[19]
Direct injury, stretching, or 2° to scar formation	Rhodes, 1957;[20] Peterson, 1952[21]
Iliac graft harvest	Mandić, 1982;[16] Massey, 1980[22]
Seat belt trauma	Beresford, 1971[23] Mandić, 1982[16]
Anomalies of passage, i.e., through the sartorius muscle	Ghent, 1961[7]
Tight girdle/clothing	Bora and Ostermann, 1982[11]
Obesity	Mandić, 1982[16]

and compression in the fascia lata and inguinal ligament. Local application of anesthetics and corticosteroids may bring immediate relief in the lower form of the syndrome. At the same time, this injection serves in the differential diagnosis. Conversative therapies for the lower form of compression include histamine therapy, ionophoresis, and use of anesthetic ointment on the affected skin. Mandić[16] recommended local anesthetics, weight loss in obese patients, optimal diabetic control, removal of compressive garments, and physical or electric therapies (i.e., electrical stimulation for analgesia, TENS). If conservative therapy fails, neurolysis or nerve resection is indicated, since patients prefer hypesthesia to burning pain.

REFERENCES

1. Roth, V. K., *Meralgia Paresthetica,* Karger, Berlin, 1895.
2. Bernhard, M., *Zentralbl. Neurol.,* 14, 242, 1895.
3. Freud, S., *Zentralbl. Neurol.,* 14, 491, 1895.
4. Mumenthaler, M. and Schliack H., *Läsionen peripherer Nerven,* G. Thieme, Stuttgart, 1965.
5. Stevens, H., *Arch. Neurol. Psychiatr.,* 77, 557, 1957.
6. Ghent, W. R., *Can. Med. Assoc. J.,* 81, 631, 1959.
7. Ghent, W. R., *Can. Med. Assoc. J.,* 85, 871, 1961.
8. Komar, J., *Alagut-szindromak,* Medicina Könyvkiado, Budapest, 1977.
9. Kopell, H. P. and Thompson, W. A. L., *Peripheral Entrapment Neuropathies,* William and Wilkins Co., Baltimore, 1963.

10. Nathan, H. J., *Neurosurgery,* 17, 843, 1960.
11. Bora, W. F. and Ostermann, A. L., *Clin. Orthop.,* 163, 20, 1982.
12. Stevens, A. and Rosselle, N., *Electromyography,* 10, 397, 1970.
13. Sarala, P. V., Nishikara, T., and Oh, S. J., *Arch. Phys. Med. Rehabil.,* 60, 30, 1979.
14. Misoul, C., Nerve injuries and entrapment syndromes of the lower extremity, in *Principles of Orthopaedic Practice,* Dee, R., Ed., McGraw-Hill, New York, 1989.
15. Gateless, D., Cullis, P., and Ingall, R. F., *Neurology,* 33, 128, 1983.
16. Mandić, V., *Med. Jad.,* 14(2-4), 316, 1982.
17. Flowers, R. S., *Am. J. Surg.,* 116, 89, 1968.
18. Carayon, A. and Gruet, M., *Bull. Soc. Med. Afr. Noire,* 14, 37, 1969.
19. Moscona, R. R. and Hirshowitz, B., *Ann. Plast. Surg.,* 4, 161, 1980.
20. Rhodes, P., *Lancet,* 2, 831, 1957.
21. Peterson, P. H., *Am. J. Obstet. Gynecol.,* 64, 690, 1952.
22. Massey, E. W., *J. Trauma,* 20, 342, 1980.
23. Beresford, H. R., *J. Trauma,* II, 629, 1971.

ILIOINGUINAL SYNDROME

The ilioinguinal nerve can be compressed as it passes through the abdominal wall between the transversis abdominis muscle and the internal and external oblique abdomini muscles. This produces both muscular and sensory dysfunction.

ANATOMY

The ilioinguinal nerve originates from the L1 nerve root, rarely L2, and descends along the quadratus lumborum and the iliacus muscles. Piercing the transversis abdominis muscle and the internal oblique muscle, the nerve comes to run under the external oblique muscle. As it runs between the internal and external oblique muscles distal and medial to the anterior superior iliac spine, the nerve changes direction and either accompanies the spermatic cord in men or the round ligament in women, the ligamentum teres of the uterus (Figure 1). Sensory fibers branch off to innervate the skin of the scrotum in men or the skin of the labia major in women. An additional sensory branch supplies the skin over the inguinal ligament.

ETIOLOGY

Described as neuralgia by Cramer in 1933,[1] many authors have described nerve injury during surgery.[2-4] Since the ilioinguinal nerve courses through the retroperitoneal space to come anteriorly over the abdominal wall, the nerve lies at risk for compression from muscular, retroperitoneal, and renal pathology.[5] Additionally, pathology involving the spermatic cord or the round ligament may damage the nerve. Inguinal hernias may also distort the muscular tunnel. Kopell, Thompson, and Postel[6] describe the ilioinguinal syndrome as a tunnel syndrome based on the functional anatomy.

The ilioinguinal nerve has been described as being susceptible to stretching, since its length is fixed between its origin and where it pierces through the abdominal musculature at the level of the anterior superior iliac spine.[6] This muscular tunnel fixes the nerve. Therefore, dynamic or permanent changes in the position of the hip or the pelvis will create tension on the nerve. Prolonged or recurrent stretches will damage the nerve. Additionally, if hip motion and therefore gait is affected, compensatory movement can further alter abdominal muscle motion during gait. Altered abdominal movements can also compress a stretched nerve. Other investigators have noted the interdependence of osteoarthritis of the hip joint and development of the ilioinguinal syndrome.[7,8] Compression due to prolonged coughing in individuals with bronchial asthma has been postulated, as the function of the abdominal musculature has repeated stresses.

CLINICAL SYMPTOMS AND SIGNS

Patients present with pain in the inguinal region that may irradiate to the hip. Abdominal wall tension or erect posturing may increase their symptoms. Occasionally, their pain may have begun after raising a heavy weight.

Pressure medially and distal to the anterior superior iliac spine will reproduce their pain as radiation along the inguinal ligament. Sensory disturbances (hypesthesis, hypalgesia, and dysthesias) will be appreciated along the ilioinguinal dermatomes. Abdominal muscular weakness and atrophy can be appreciated by having the patient try to rise from a supine position. Contraction of the abdominal muscles will produce a protrusion of abdominal contents above the inguinal ligament. To help themselves rise, patients will pull their legs towards their body as they bend forward. Others have described a sudden crooked gait secondary to the syndrome.[6,7]

The differential diagnosis must contain retroperitoneal and renal pathologies, genitofemoral nerve damage or entrapment, and meralgia paresthetica. Occurring after inguinal hernia

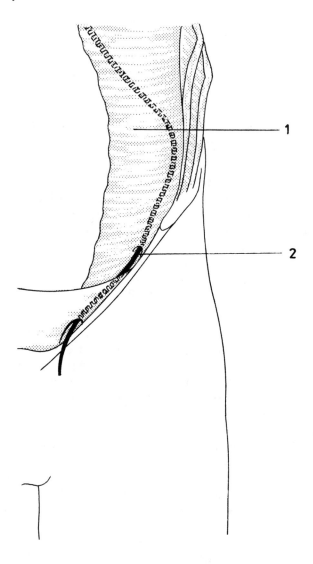

FIGURE 1.   The ilioinguinal nerve (2) lies in a susceptible position for nerve compression and damage as it pierces the transversis abdominis muscle (1) and its fascia.

repair, appendectomy, or Cesarean sections, entrapment or damage to the genitofemoral nerve creates chronic pain and paresthesias over the upper thigh distal to the femoral triangle and in the lateral scrotum or labia[9] as well as loss of the cremaster muscle reflex. One should be able to distinguish meralgia paresthetica by affected dermatome examination.

TREATMENT

Removal of compressive causes as well as those causes which place the nerve under tension are necessary to relieve the syndrome. Static changes in the hip and pelvis are more difficult to treat. However, a trial of physical therapy, local corticosteroid injection, and gait modification may be effective. If conservative therapy does not succeed, surgical therapy, which may include sectioning of the nerve, is indicated.

REFERENCES

1. Cramer, H., *Zentralbl. Gynakol.,* 57, 1966, 1933
2. Magee, R.K. *Can. Med. Assoc. J.,* 46, 236, 1942.
3. Lyon, F. K., *Can. Med. Assoc. J.,* 53, 213, 1945.
4. Bernaschek, W., *Zentralbl. Chir.,* 79, 62, 1954.
5. Stabli, R., *Praxis,* 54, 273, 1965.
6. Kopell, H. P., Thompson, W. A. L., Postel, A. H., *N. Engl. J. Med.,* 266, 16, 1962.
7. Komar, J., *Nervenarzt,* 42, 637, 1971.
8. Mumenthaler, A., Mumenthaler, M., Luciani, H., and Kramer, *J.: Dtsch. Med. Wochenschr.,* 90, 1073, 1965.
9. Harms, B. A., DeHass, D. R., and Starling, J. R., *Arch. Surg.,* 119, 339, 1984.

SAPHENOUS NERVE SYNDROME

The saphenous nerve passes through the adductor canal and penetrates the vasto-adductor membrane to run superficially (Figure 1). Compression or stretching of the nerve in this area produces pain along its dermatomes.

NATOMY

The anatomical relations of this canal have been studied by Jo and Solter.[1] The longest sensory branch of the femoral nerve, the saphenous nerve, leaves the femoral triangle to enter the adductor canal together with the femoral artery and vein. The vastus medialis muscle and adductor longus muscle, the canal's walls, are connected by a vasto-adductor membrane, the canal's roof. The sartorius muscle also covers the proximal portion of the canal and later covers the two terminal branches of the saphenous nerve, the infrapatellar and the descending branches.

The infrapatellar branch bends at 90° to the longitudinal axis of the femur at the level of the knee's joint line. Sending a branch between the superficial and deep layers of the medial collateral ligament, the infrapatellar branch supplies the medial portion of the joint and the overlying skin. This small branch may be injured in surgery or meniscal dislocation. The descending branch accompanies the saphenous vein to supply the skin of the medial leg and foot.

ETIOLOGY

Extensively studied by many investigators,[2-5] trauma along the adductor canal or vasto-adductor membrane underlies most of the described etiologies. Mumenthaler and Schliack[6] and Jones[7] described saphenous nerve damage in association with femoral arteriography and vascular surgery, respectively. Inflammatory disorders like saphenous vein thrombophlebitis may reduce the space within the canal and lead to compression. However, trauma predominates, since surgery around the knee menisectomy, arthrotomy,[8] ligament reconstruction, arthroscopy, and knee arthroplasty) and saphenous vein (surgery for varicosities) has increased in recent times.[9,10] Direct trauma to the canal in sports like soccer or rugby can damage the nerve.

Functional anatomy has been used to explain nerve compression. Kopell and Thompson[11] described that changes in knee position (especially genu varum), deformation with torsion, or direct trauma due to trauma lead to stretching and mechanical irritation of the nerve in the region of the vasto-adductor membrane. Dumitru and Windsor[12] have described subsartorial entrapment in a body builder.

CLINICAL SYMPTOMS AND SIGNS

Patients present with constant medial leg pain when walking and climbing, leading to possible confusion of this syndrome with vascular disorders.[13] Pressure over the adductor canal or where the nerve crosses the medial femoral condyle produces strong pain radiating down to the medial malleolus. Physical examination typically reveals hyperalgesia and hyperesthesia in the infrapatellar region and hypalgesia and hypesthesia along the medial leg and foot. Resisted adduction produces pain in the canal.[11] Pain with knee hyperextension leads patients to walk without fully extending their knees. This altered gait loads the foot abnormally and may lead to the development of metatarsalgia.[11]

Pain relief despite provocation, following a local novocaine injection into the adductor canal, may isolate this syndrome.[14] Occasionally, injury to the infrapatellar branch occurs simultaneously with medial meniscal damage producing Turner's symptom of hypesthesia. As Mandi and Kalmar[15] found, 4.2% of all arthrotomies for suspected meniscal tears were found to have saphenous nerve compression instead of meniscal tear. Therefore, in the cases where a torn meniscus is questionable, one may consider testing with local novocaine injections into the canal for diagnostic confirmation.

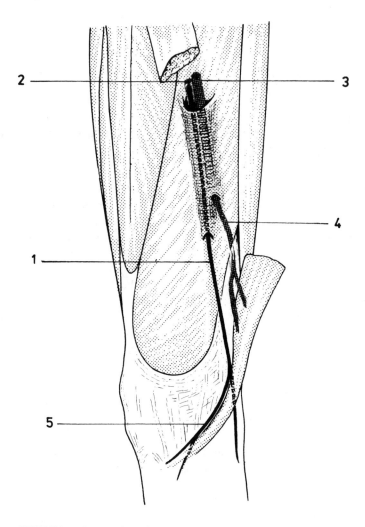

FIGURE 1.   Compression of the saphenous nerve typically occurs in the region depicted above.
1: Saphenous nerve; 2: femoral vein; 3:femoral artery; 4: descending genicular artery; 5: infrapatellar branch of the saphenous nerve.

TREATMENT

Conservative therapy is often sufficient. These measures include the following: rest, physiotherapy, anti-inflammatory medication, and local corticosteroid injection. Surgical treatment consists of sectioning of the vasto-adductor membrane from the site of compression proximally. If the sartorius muscle's tendon compresses the infrapatellar branch, the tendon may need to be partially released. While surgical exploration and neurolysis may be necessary initially, recurrent symptoms may require saphenous nerve resection.[16]

REFERENCES

1. Jo, A. and Solter, D., *Rad. Med. Fak. Zagreb,* 16, 21, 1968.
2. Lee, B. Y., Lapointe, D. G., and Madden, J. L., *Am. J. Surg.,* 123, 617, 1972.
3. Balaji, M. R. and DeWeese, J. A., *JAMA,* 245, 167, 1981.
4. Verta, M. J., Vigello, J., and Fuller, J., *Arch Surg.,* 119, 345, 1984.
5. Romanoff, M. E., Cory, C. P., Kalenak, A., Keyser, C. G., and Marshall, K. W., *Am. J. Sports Med.,* 17, 478, 1989.
6. Mumenthaler, M. and Schliack, H., *Läsionen peripherer Nerven,* G. Thieme, Stuttgart, 1965.
7. Jones, N. A., *Br. J. Surg.,* 65, 465, 1978.
8. Chambers, G. H., *Clin. Orthop.,* 82, 157, 1972.
9. Komar, J., *Alagut-szindromak,* Medicina Könyvkiado, Budapest, 1957.
10. Fischer, R., *Helv. Chir. Acta,* 28, 168, 1961.
11. Kopell, H. P. and Thompson, W. A. L., *N. Engl. J. Med.,* 263, 351, 1963.
12. Dumitru, D. and Windsor, R. E., *Phys. Sports Med.,* 17, 116, 1989.
13. Mozes, M., Quaknine, G., and Nathan, H., *Surgery,* 77, 299, 1975.
14. Meier, W., *Z. Unfallmed. Berufskr.,* 63, 129, 1970.
15. Mandi, A. and Kalmar, L., *Orv. Hetil,* 114, 925, 1973.
16. Luerssen, T. G., Campbell, R. L., Defalque, R. J., and Worth, R. M., *Neurosurgery,* 13, 238, 1983.

POPLITEAL ENTRAPMENT SYNDROME

The tendinous arch of the soleus muscle and the popliteus muscle delineate the popliteal fossa, through which pass the popliteal artery vein and the tibial nerve (Figure 1). In contrast to the remainder of syndromes in this book, the tibial nerve does not get compressed in the popliteal fossa. Limited data exist in the medical literature concerning neurovascular compression of the popliteal artery in this region, which has been described as either popliteal artery entrapment syndrome[1] or popliteal entrapment syndrome. In 1959, Hamming[2] focused attention on it by describing an intraoperative finding in a patient with intermittent claudication. The most frequent causes of arterial compression are anatomical variations of the popliteal artery or the muscles crossing the fossa. Described originally in 1879 by Stuart,[3] these variations convert the popliteal fossa into a tunnel.

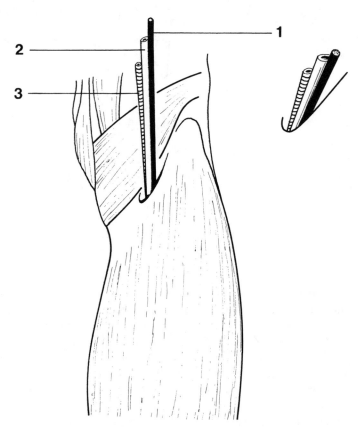

FIGURE 1.   This figure illustrates the typical relationship of the popliteal artery (3), the popliteal vein (2), and the tibial nerve (1) as they course ove the popliteus muscle and under the medial head of the gastrochemius muscle.

ANATOMY

Continuing the femoral artery's course after leaving the opening in the adductor magnus muscle tendon, the popliteal artery angles towards the lateral side of the fossa, reaches the middle of the fossa midway through the fossa, and then courses distally between the medial and lateral

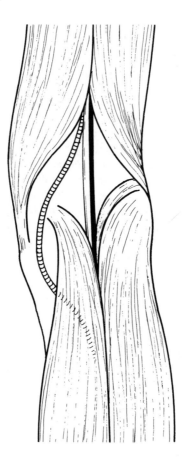

FIGURE 2.   This figure shows an anom-
aly in the popliteal artery as it courses
around the medial head of the gastrochemius muscle.

heads of the gastrocnemius muscle to dive under the tendinous arch of the soleus muscle. The
popliteal artery divides into the anterior and posterior tibial arteries after crossing the tendinous
arch. The popliteal artery lies deep to the popliteal vein and deep and medial to the tibial nerve
in the fossa. The artery lies in close approximation to the popliteal surface of the fossa, the knee
joint capsule, and the posterior surface of the popliteus muscle. The popliteal fossa is bounded
as follows: laterally by the biceps femoris, proximally by the plantaris, distally by the lateral head
of the gastrocnemius, and medially by the semitendinosus, semimembranosus, and the medial
head of the gastrocnemius; "the roof is covered by the fascia lata."[4] While these are the classic
relationships, variations do arise.

Stuart[3] and Hamming[2] described arteries, which instead of passing between the heads of the
gastrocneomicus, passed between the medial head of the gastrocnemius and the medial femoral
condyle. The muscle head's proximal origin is due to embryonal development. Chambardel-
Dubreuil[5] described an artery coursing through the medial head (Figure 2). These variations
place the artery at risk for intermittent compression with muscle activity. The popliteal vein may
follow the artery's anomalous course.[6]

ETIOLOGY

Many investigators describe intermittent claudication associated with a popliteal artery that
is compressed between the gastrocnemius and medial femoral condyle or by the gastrocnemius

TABLE 1
The Modified Classification of Popliteal Artery Entrapment

Type	Muscle	Artery	Associated vessels
I	Normal	Anomalous course	None
Ia	Proximal origin	Minimally displaced	None
II	Aberrant origin or accessory head	Normal	None
IIa	Medially placed plantaris joins the medial head	Normal	None

tendinous origin itself.[7,8] Based on these varied relationships, Insua et al.[9] classified the anomalies into four categories, which have since been modified: in Type I, the artery passes along the internal margin of the normal medial head of the gastrocnemius before turning over the margin to reach the fossa from under the muscles's head; in Type Ia, the medial head of the gastrocnemius originates more proximally on the femur, thus covering the minimally displaced popliteal artery; in Type II, the gastrocnemius has an accessory head or aberrant tendinous bundle, lateral to the medial head, which covers a nondisplaced popliteal artery; and in Type IIa, a medially placed plantaris unites with the medial head of the gastrocnemius over normal popliteal artery. The modifications have been made by multiple investigators describing over 160 cases on entrapment (see Table 1).[10-14] Becquemin et al.[14] emphasize the possibility of compression due to anomalies in the semimembranosus, semitendinosus, adductor magnus, or tendinous arch of the soleus. However, the tendinous arch is only mentioned as a possibility. Compression by the arch would compress the popliteal artery and vein and the tibial nerve, providing a neurologic presentation of the popliteal entrapment syndrome.

CLINICAL SYMPTOMS AND SIGNS

Popliteal entrapment syndrome should be suspected in young, active patients who present with intermittent claudication. Their clinical picture depends on the presence of thromboses, aneurysms, or only dynamic compression with activities.

Ischemic symptoms may involve only the foot or the entire leg. Since nerves are the most sensitive tissue, ischemia leads to numbness, tingling, and feelings of cold, pain, and paresthesia. The leg muscles can cramp intermittently. Claudication remains the most constant symptom. The other symptoms may develop only after intensive exercises or just after walking but not running. Weakening or disappearance of the dorsalis pedis pulse with maximal dorsiflexion or plantar flexion with an extended knee implicates popliteal artery compression. Relief of symptoms and reappearance of the arterial pulse with rest strengthen the argument for compression. Thromboses or aneurysms of the popliteal artery may lead to acute ischemic attacks or emboli, which are more severe than the temporary ischemic changes of cramps and sensory dysfunction.[6,13-18]

Invasive and noninvasive vascular exams aid in diagnosis. Doppler ultrasound allows dynamic arterial testing during active muscular contraction in plantar flexion and dorsiflexion. Impedance plethysmography evaluates ankle, calf, and thigh pressures and pulses and can be used in conjunction with treadmill tests. Appearance of symptoms during testing confirms the suspicion. The combination of all the data from these tests differentiates popliteal entrapment syndrome from peripheral vascular disease, neurogenic claudication, psychoneurosis, and anterior compartment syndrome. Bell[18] advocated the use of compartment pressure measurements to clearly define patients with presumed compartment syndrome, McDonald et al.[16]

recommended angiography to detail medial dislocation (i.e., behind the medial femoral condyle), and selective biplane angiography (anteroposterior, lateral) with changes in foot position from dorsiflexion, to neutral, and then to plantar flexion. Maximal dorsiflexion may require assistance. Arterial narrowing or obliteration may occur with popliteal entrapment syndrome.

TREATMENT

Surgical decompression may require maneuvers that do not affect muscle function, e.g., decompression of the artery by dividing the compressive structures and resection of the damaged arterial segment. The segment may be replaced by a saphenous vein graft or repaired by performing an endarterectomy. If the artery is normal, removal of the compressive agent is sufficient.

REFERENCES

1. Love, J. W. and Whelan, T. J., *Am. J. Surg.,* 109, 620, 1965.
2. Hamming, J. J., *Angiology,* 10, 369, 1959.
3. Stuart, T. P. A., *J. Anat. Physiol.,* 13, 162, 1879.
4. Gray, H., *Anatomy of the Human Body,* Lea & Febigner, Philadelphia, 1973.
5. Chambardel-Dubreuil, L., *Variation des artéres du Pelvis et du Membre Inférieur,* Masson, Paris, 1925.
6. Gibson, M. H. L., Mills, M. S., Johnson, G. E., and Downs, A. R., *Ann. Surg.,* 185, 341, 1977.
7. Servello, M., *Circulation,* 26, 885, 1962.
8. Carter, A. E. and Eban, R., *Br. J. Surg.,* 51, 518, 1964.
9. Insua, J. A., Young, J. R., and Humphires, A. W., *Arch. Surg.,* 101, 771, 1970.
10. Rich, N. M. and Hughes, C. W., *Am. J. Surg.,* 113, 696, 1965.
11. Delaney, T. A. and Gonzalez, L. L., *Surgery,* 69, 97, 1971.
12. Ferrero, R., Barile, D., Buzzacchino, A., Bretto, P., and Ponzio, F., *Minerva Cardiangiol.,* 26, 389, 1978.
13. Rich, N. M., Collins, G. J., McDonald, P. T., Kozloff, L., Clagett, P., and Collins, J. T., *Arch. Surg.,* 114, 1377, 1979.
14. Becquemin, J. P., Melléire, D., Lamour, A., and Kenesi, C., *Ant. Clin.,* 6, 203, 1984.
15. Darlin, R. C., Buckley, C. J., Abbot, W. M., and Raines, J. K., *J. Trauma,* 14, 543, 1974.
16. McDonald, P. T., Easterbrook, J. A., Rich, M. N., Collins, G. J., Kozloff, L., Clagett, G. P., and Collins, J. T., *Am. J. Surg.,* 139, 318, 1980.
17. Ikeda, M., Iwase, T., Ashida, K., and Tankawa, J. H., *Am. J. Surg.,* 141, 726, 1981.
18. Bell, S., *Am. J. Sports Med.,* 13, 365, 1985.

PERONEAL TUNNEL SYNDROME

The common peroneal nerve runs in an exposed fibro-osseus tunnel at the level of the fibular neck. Compression produces a characteristic clinical picture which, while it bears many names in the medical literature (restless legs, crossed legs palsy, isolated peroneal nerve palsy at the head of the fibula), will be discussed here as the peroneal tunnel syndrome.

ANATOMY

The common peroneal nerve usually branches from the sciatic nerve in the proximal portion of the popliteal fossa. Variations occur where the nerve leaves proximally or distally.[1] The nerve runs along the biceps femoris muscle and tendon to the popliteal fossa (Figure 1). The nerve then encircles the head of the fibula, passes below the tendinous origin of the peroneus longus and enters the peroneal tunnel near the fibular neck (Figure 2). Proximal to the fibular head, the lateral sural cutaneous nerve branches from the common peroneal nerve.

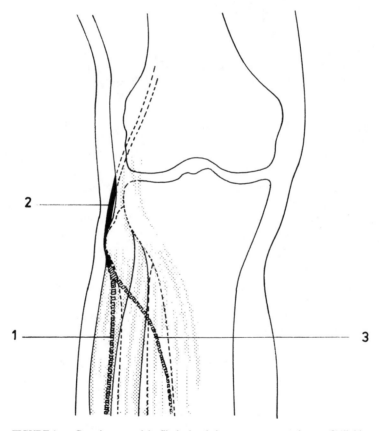

FIGURE 1.   Coursing around the fibular head, the common peroneal nerve (2) divides into a superficial (1) and a deep (profundus, 3) branch. The deep branch dives deep to run along the intercompartmental fascial plane.

As the nerve enters the tunnel, the common peroneal nerve divides into the deep, superficial, and recurrent peroneal nerves. Additional branches to the peroneus longus and anterior tibialis muscles may be found at the tunnel's entrance. Bogdanović et al.[2] described branch points at the

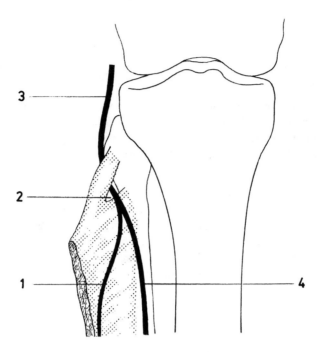

FIGURE 2.   Occasionally the common peroneal nerve (3) or one of its branches (the superficial (1) or the deep branch (4)) can be compressed by the tendinous arch of the peroneus longus muscle (2).

level of fibular neck in 67% of the cases, at the level of the fibular head in 22% of the cases, and more proximal in the popliteal fossa in 11% of the cases.

In the peroneal tunnel, the peroneal nerve and its branches stretch over the periosteum of the fibular neck and are covered by the tendinous origin of the peroneus longus muscle. This tendinous origin can be found in the shape of a hook or J on the left leg or reversed J on the right leg.[3] Plantar flexion or foot inversion (adduction, supination, and plantar flexion) tenses the peroneus longus muscle and brings it closer to the fibula. This motion decreases the tunnel's space and compresses the nerve against the fibular neck. The deep and the superficial branches are stretched and bend over the lower hook of the tendinous arch.

The superficial peroneal nerve (superficialis peroneus) runs between the fibula and the peroneus longus muscle. As it courses distally, it lies on the anterior intermuscular septum between either the peroneus longus muscle proximally and the extensor digitorum longus muscle, or (distally) and the peroneus longus muscle, the peroneus brevis muscle. The superficial peroneal nerve supplies both the peroneus brevis and longus muscles. At the junction of the middle and distal third of the tibia, the superficial peroneal nerve pierces the crural fascia and splits into two cutaneous branches. Compression by the crural fascia produces the syndrome of the superficial peroneal nerve. The terminal branches, the medial dorsal cutaneous pedal and the intermediate dorsal cutaneous pedal branches, supply the anterolateral skin of the leg and the dorsal skin of the great, second, third, and medial fourth toes. The dorsum of the lateral fourth and the fifth toes are innervated by the sural nerve via the lateral dorsal cutaneous pedal nerve.

Dividing from the common peroneal nerve, the deep peroneal nerve (peroneus profundus) pierces the anterior intermuscular septum and travels with the anterior tibial vessel between the tibialis anterior muscle and either the extensor digitorum longus muscle proximally or the extensor hallucis longus muscle distally. In this fashion, these muscles receive their innervation from the deep peroneal nerve. The nerve enters the foot under the cruciform ligament (anterior tarsal tunnel syndrome), provides dorsum of the articular branches, and ends in the first metatarsal space with sensory branches to the skin between the great and the second toes.

TABLE 1
Etiologies and Investigators for Peroneal Tunnel Syndrome

Etiology	Investigator
External	
Plaster casts (short leg, PTBs)	Mumenthaler, 1973[6]
Crossed legs (prolonged)	Woltmann, 1929[7]
	Nagler and Rangel, 1947[8]
	Marwah, 1967[9]
Sleeping positions	Bora and Osterman, 1982[10]
Unknown	
Idiopathic	Osborne, 1957;[11] Fettweis, 1968;[12]
Repetitive trauma	Kopell and Thompson, 1960;[3] Moller and
(functional anatomy)	Kadin, 1987 (runners);[13] Leach et al., 1989
	(runners)[14]]
Internal	
Bony changes	
(a) exostosis	Theodorou et al., 1978[15]
(b) osteophyte	Sheman et al., 1983[16]
(c) fibular fractures	Casselt and Dürrschmidt, 1969;[17] Komar, 1977[18]
Knee arthroplasty	Rose et al., 1982[4]
Ganglions	Brooks, 1952;[19] Parkes, 1961;[20] Clark, 1961;[21]
	Muckart, 1976;[22] Bora and Osterman, 1982[10]
Synovial cysts	Kopell and Thompson, 1963[3]
Other	
(a) Hemophiliac	Large et al., 1983[23]
(b) enlarged fabella	Mangieri, 1973[24]

ETIOLOGY

Compression in the area of the peroneal tunnel frequently comes from an external source, as shown in Table 1. These external causes can be as simple as a short leg cast tightly placed with the knee in hyperextension. The close relationship of the common peroneal nerve to the fibula places it at risk with fibular fractures or correction of valgus knees during knee arthroplasty.[4] Synovial cysts or ganglions can displace the nerve from its course and place it into a prolonged stretch.[5] The cysts can actually enter into the tunnel and directly compress the nerve. While idiopathic forms still exist, many previously idiopathic cases may be explained by functional anatomical changes. Repetitive actions requiring inversion or pronation (e.g., runners and machine operators using pedals) stretch the common peroneal nerve against the fibula and the lower margin of the tendinous arch. The concurrent weakness in dorsiflexion and eversion as well as sensory complaints may be confused with chronic subtalar synovitis or chronic talar subluxations.

CLINICAL SYMPTOMS AND SIGNS

Pain appears initially in the compressed region before spreading distally into the common peroneal nerve's dermatome, which includes the dermatomes of the deep and the superficial peroneal nerves. Radiation of pain into the thigh may occur. Additional palpation or pressure over the tunnel will increase the patient's pain. This pain will not be felt in lumbar stenosis, root entrapment, or more proximal compression. Presenting gradually after the appearance of lateral leg and dorsal foot pain, motor weakness and atrophy can lead to a full-blown dropped-foot presentation. Patients will have weakness on dorsiflexion and inversion. Forced inversion will actually increase their pain. Trophic changes in the bones of the foot may occur with neural dysfunction. Electromyographic and nerve conduction velocity studies will aid in differentiating peroneal tunnel syndrome from sciatica, lumbar stenosis, syndrome of the piriformis muscle, polyneuropathies, and anterior tibial syndrome. Close examination of the dermatomes involved greatly helps. If compression occurs proximal to the thigh, other nerve areas including the tibial nerve may be involved. In the piriformis muscle syndrome, pain is localized to the gluteal region without reproduction of pain with peroneal tunnel palpation. Conduction velocity studies will verify normal conduction across the peroneal tunnel if nerve compression is occurring proximally. Patients with anterior tibial syndrome will typically present with a swollen red leg, strong pain, and a missing dorsalis pedis arterial pulse. The pain in polyneuropathies is sharp, burning, and independent of motion, with electromyographic studies implicating the spinal cord as the source. The sensory changes are circular and the leg is hypotonic without reflexes but with trophic skin changes.

TREATMENT

Identification of a specific peroneal tunnel syndrome's etiology allows appropriate treatment. External compressive causes must be relieved. Repetitive motions that irritate the nerve must be avoided. Local corticosteroid injections may bring relief. Physical therapy allows strengthening of atrophied muscles following either conservative or surgical relief of nerve compression. Failure of conservative therapy to relieve the symptoms necessitates surgical decompression of the tunnel.

REFERENCES

1. Pećina, M., *Oβtecenja zivcanog stabla i ogranaka ishijadikusa uvjetovana posebnim topografsko-anatomskim odnosima,* disertacija, Medicinski fakultet, Zagreb, 1970.
2. Bogdanović, D., Ilić, A., and Marenić, S., *Acta Orthop. Lugosl.,* 3, 357, 1972.
3. Kopell, H. P. and Thompson, W. A. L., *N. Engl. J. Med.,* 262, 56, 1960.
4. Rose, H. A., Hood, R. W., Otis, J. C., et al., *J. Bone Joint Surg.,* 64A, 347, 1982.
5. Tupmann, G. S., *Br. J. Surg.,* 45, 23, 1957.
6. Mumenthaler, M., *Schweiz. Arch. Neurol. Neurochir. Psychiatr.,* 112, 229, 1973.
7. Woltmann, H. W., *JAMA,* 93, 670, 1929.
8. Nagler, S. H. and Rangel, L., *JAMA,* 133, 755, 1947.
9. Marwah, V., *Lancet,* 2, 367, 1967.
10. Bora, F. W. and Osterman, A. L., *Clin. Orthop.,* 163, 20, 1982.
11. Osborne, G. V., *J. Bone Joint Surg.,* 39B, 782, 1957.
12. Fettweis, E., *Dtsch. Med. Wochenschr.,* 93, 1393, 1968.
13. Moller, B. N. and Kadin, S., *Am. J. Sports Med.,* 15, 90, 1987.
14. Leach, R. E., Purnell, B. M., and Saito, A., *Am. J. Sports Med.,* 17, 287, 1989.
15. Theodorou, S. D., Karamitosos, S., Tsouparopolulos, D., and Hatzipavlou, A. G., *Acta Orthop. Belg.,* 44, 496, 1978.
16. Sheman, O., Testa, N. N., and Klein, M. J., *Orthopedics,* 6, 1317, 1983.
17. Casselt, C. and Durrschmidt, V., *Beitr. Orthop. Trauma,* 16, 444, 1969.
18. Komar, J., *Alagut-szindromak,* Medicina Könyvkiado, Budapest, 1977.
19. Brooks, D. M., *J. Bone Joint Surg.,* 34B, 391, 1952.
20. Parkes, A., *J. Bone Joint Surg.,* 43B, 784, 1961.
21. Clark, K., *J. Bone Joint Surg.,* 43B, 788, 1961.
22. Muckart, R. O., *J. Bone Joint Surg.,* 58B, 241, 1976.
23. Large, D. F., Ludlam, C. A., and MacNicol, M. F., *Clin. Orthop.,* 181(1), 65, 1983.
24. Mangieri, J. V., *J. Bone Joint Surg.,* 55A, 395, 1973.

SUPERFICIAL PERONEAL NERVE SYNDROME

Compression or distortion of the superficial peroneal nerve may occur where the nerve abandons the muscular layer of the leg and pierces the crural fascia at the level between the middle and distal third of the leg. The syndrome of the superficial peroneal nerve was first described in 1945 by Henry[1] under the term *mononeuralgia in the superficial peroneal nerve* and is also known recently as *superficial peroneal nerve entrapment*.

ANATOMY

At the entrance into the peroneal tunnel near the head of the fibula, the common peroneal nerve divides into two terminal branches, the deep and superficial peroneal nerve (Figure 1). This terminal branch point may vary as well as the superficial peroneal nerve's course. The superficial branch continues distally between the fibula and the peroneus longus muscle lying on the intermuscular septum of the anterior compartment. The nerve also lies between the peroneus longus and the extensor digitorum longus muscles proximally and the peroneus longus and brevis muscles distally. At the level between the middle and distal thirds of the leg, the nerve pierces the crural fascia and continues subcutaneously as the cutaneous dorsalis medialis and the cutaneous dorsalis intermedius nerves. Prior to piercing the fascia, the superficial peroneal nerve supplies the peroneus longus and brevis muscles. The cutaneous branches of the superficial nerves supply the skin of the anterolateral side of the leg, the dorsum of the foot, the dorsum of the first, second, and third toes, and the medial side of the fourth toe. The sural nerve via the cutaneous dorsalis lateralis nerve supplies the lateral sides of the fourth and fifth toes.

ETIOLOGY

Trauma represents the most common proposed etiolgy of the rarely diagnosed syndrome of the superficial peroneal nerve.[2-4] Surgical trauma, lipomas,[5] muscular hernias,[6,7] tight boots,[5] repetitive compression at the foot in sports,[8] and dynamic compression in the narrow fascial tunnel[1,2,5] have been postulated as etiologies. Styf and Korner[9] and Styf[10] have described the development of the syndrome after fasciotomy for chronic anterior compartment syndrome. Traume in this area may lead to local inflammation and reactive swelling, and eventually compression in the fascial tunnel.

Dynamic compression based on the functional anatomy of the leg places the nerve at risk.[11,12] The superficial peroneal nerve is fixed; therefore, forced inversion and extension of the foot further stretches the nerve over the fascial border.[1,2,5] Surgical data revealed marked narrowing in 12 or 19 subjects, poststenotic edema in 5 or 19 subjects, and muscular hernia in the tunnel in 6 of 19 subjects.[10] While typically noted as 1 cm in length, surgical evidence showed that the tunnel may actuallly run 3 to 11 cm in length (10 of 19 subjects).[10] Repetitive activities may cause scarring of the nerve or fascial borders, further narrowing the tunnel.

CLINICAL SYMPTOMS AND SIGNS

Described as mononeuralgia in 1945 by Henry,[1] pain caused by compression or damage to the superficial peroneal nerve appears on the dorsum of the foot accompanied sometimes by dysesthesias or complete anesthesia in the nerve's dermatome (Figure 2). Styf[10] suggested three tests for evaluating patients for the syndrome: first, resisted dorsiflexion and eversion with pressure applied over the tunnel; second, passive plantar flexion and inversion; and third, stretching of the nerve as in the second test with percussion over the tunnel. A positive result for these provocative tests is the production of pain or parathesias over the nerve's dermatome. Electromyographic studies of the peroneal and anterior tibial muscles and conduction velocity examination help in identifying the syndrome. Radiographic examination will help to eliminate

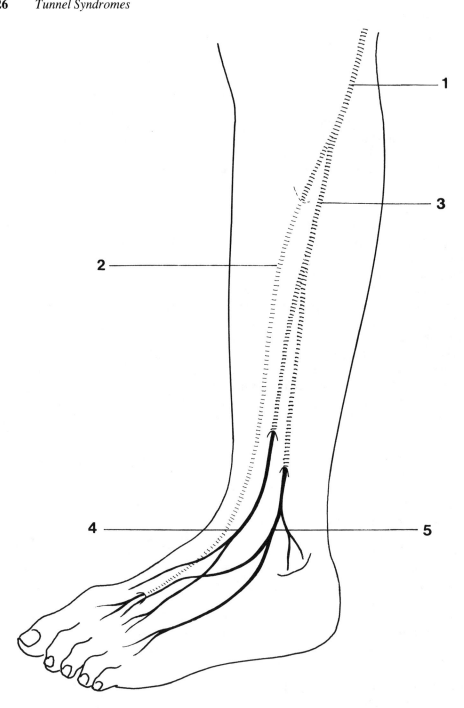

FIGURE 1.   This figure details the relationship of the peroneal nerves as they reach the foot.
1: Common peroneal nerve; 2: deep peroneal nerve; 3: superficial peroneal nerve; 4: medial dorsal
cutaneous nerve; 5 intermediate dorsal cutaneous nerve; deep peroneal nerve.

other pathological states in the area such as stress fractures or tumors. Since lumbosacral spine
pathology can easily involve various nerve roots, one should not be misled and jump to
conclusions when presented with lower extremity neurological symptoms. Bannerjee and
Koons[1] described a case of superficial peroneal compression treated only after L4/5 discectomy

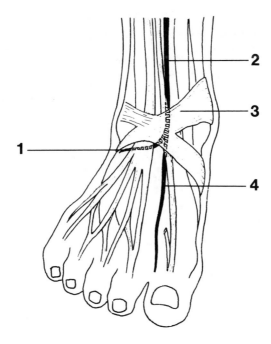

FIGURE 2.   The deep peroneal nerve may be compressed as it enters the dorsum of the foot under the extensor retinaculum.
1: Lateral branch of the deep peroneal nerve; 2: deep peroneal nerve; 3: inferior extensor retinaculum (cruciform ligament); 4: medial branch of the deep peroneal nerve.

failed to resolve an individual's pain. An invasive but diagnostic test using local injection of anasthetic over the tunnel will temporarily relieve pain due to compression in the tunnel.

TREATMENT

Since trauma ranks as a common etiology, removal of trauma should be included in the treatment protocol. Many of the movements that stretch the nerve, however, are among normal daily activities. Therefore, conservative therapy may not succeed. Passive changes in the foot's position may be beneficial. Physical therapy and local corticosteroid injections at the fascial tunnel may also be effective. If these fail to relieve the symptoms, fasciotomy of the nerve's tunnel should free the nerve and give lasting results.

REFERENCES

1. Henry, A. K., *Extensile Exposure,* E. and S. Livingston, Edinburgh-London, 1945, 296.
2. Kopell, H. P. and Thompson, W. A. L., *Peripheral Entrapment Neuropathies,* Williams and Wilkins, Baltimore, 1963.
3. Stack, R. E., Branco, A. J. Jr., and McCarty, C. S., *J. Bone Joint Surg.,* 47A, 773, 1965.
4. Tibrewal, S. B. and Goodfellow, J. W., *J. R. Soc. Med.,* 77, 72, 1984.
5. Bannerjee, T. and Koons, D. D., *J. Neurosurg.,* 55, 991, 1981.
6. Garfin, S., Mubarak, S. J., and Owen, A., *J. Bone Joint Surg.,* 59A, 404, 1977.
7. McAuliffe, T. B., Fiddian, N. J., and Browett, J. P., *J. Bone Joint Surg.,* 67B, 62, 1985.

8. Sabetta, E., *Int. J. Sports Traumatol.,* 11, 65, 1989.
9. Styf, J. R. and Korner, I., *J. Bone Joint Surg.,* 68A, 1338, 1986.
10. Styf, J. R., *J. Bone Joint Surg.,* 71B, 131, 1989.
11. Kernohan, J., Levack, B., and Wilson, J. N., *J. Bone Joint Surg.,* 67B, 60, 1985.
12. Lowdon, I., *J. Bone Joint Surg.,* 67B, 58, 1985.

ANTERIOR TARSAL TUNNEL SYNDROME
(SYNDROME OF THE ANTERIOR TARSAL CANAL;
SYNDROME OF THE DEEP PERONEAL NERVE)

When passing under the inferior extensor retinaculum (ligamentum cruciforme) on the dorsum of the foot, the deep peroneal nerve (peroneus profundus) can be compressed resulting in pain through the dermatome, which receives branches originating distal to the retinaculum. Marinacci described the clinical symptoms of the anterior tarsal tunnel syndrome in detail.[1]

ANATOMY

The anterior tarsal tunnel lies under a thickening of the dorsalis pedis fascia and above the talus bone. These fascial thickenings form a retinaculum that fixes and redirects the extensor tendons. While at times consisting of four branches in a cruciform shape, the inferior extensor retinaculum typically has three branches forming a letter **Y** transversely across the foot's dorsum. The base of the **Y**, the lateral portion, originates in the sinus tarsi on the lateral side of the calcaneus. As it passes over the tendons for the extensor digitorum longus, the retinaculum divides into two rami: the superior ramus, which inserts on the medial malleolus and the inferior ramus, which inserts on the dorsal surface of the navicular and first cuneiform bones. Occasionally, a superfluous second lateral branch may exist, which inserts on the lateral malleolus, producing a retinaculum with a cruciform shape, the ligamentum cruciforme. Medially and below the superior and inferior rami, the tendons and the tendon sheaths of the anterior tibialis and extensor hallucis longus muscles run accompanied by the dorsalis pedis artery and vein. The deep peroneal nerve joins these structures in the anterior tarsal tunnel after innervating all the foot extensor except for the extensor digitorum brevis muscle, which is the only muscle affected by anterior tarsal tunnel compression. Within the tunnel, the nerve divides into a lateral and a medial branch (Figure 1).

The lateral branch passes under the tendon of the extensor digitorum brevis muscle to innervate the tarsal and metatarsal joints via articular branches. Passing under the tendon of the extensor hallucis brevis muscle, the medial branch continues distally to terminate in the space between the great toe, and the second toe supplying sensory innervation via the dorsalis hallucis lateralis nerve and the second medial digital nerve.

ETIOLOGY

Anatomical relationships play a major role in the development of anterior tarsal tunnel syndrome. The tunnel consists of a tight retinaculum overlying mobile soft-tissue structures that lie in close approximation to the bony floor. This tight band fixes the structures. Therefore, bony, joint, vascular, neural, or muscular disorders will alter the tunnel's volume. The soft tissue structures in the tunnel act distal to the tunnel. Therefore, sudden movement or repetitive actions far from the tunnel can stretch and damage the nerve.[2] Distortion of the talonavicular joint or underlying bony surface by osteophytes, synovial pseudocysts, ganglions, and fractures compress the tunnel.[1-5] Repetitive compressive trauma from shoe straps and prolonged stretching from the prolonged plantar flexion of high-heeled shoes have been postulated as etiologies.[1,6,7] Inflammation of the tendons or development of tendon sheath or retinaculum ganglions may also narrow the tunnel. Lastly, primary neurovascular diseases such as neuromas or aneurysms may decrease the tunnel's volume.

CLINICAL SYMPTOMS AND SIGNS

The clinical picture varies depending on whether the sensory or motor fibers of the deep peroneal nerve are affected. Characteristic of sensory compromise, burning pain will be localized to the dorsal space between the great and the second toes. Blunt undefined pain felt deep in the foot coexists with disturbed extensor digitorum brevis muscle function when the

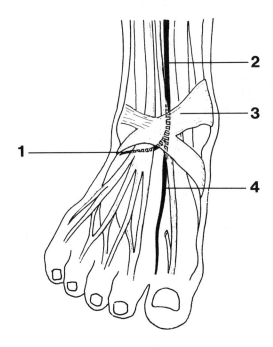

FIGURE 1.   The deep peroneal nerve may be compressed as it enters the dorsum of the foot under the extensor retinaculum.

1: Lateral branch of the deep peroneal nerve; 2: deep peroneal nerve; 3: inferior extensor retinaculum (cruciform ligament); 4: medial branch of the deep peroneal nerve.

motor fibers are compressed. Trophic changes of the metatarsal bones (i.e., osteoporosis) may occur with motor fiber compromise. To assess extensor digitorum brevis muscle function, the foot is maximally dorsiflexed, eliminating the action of the long extensor. Then the patient is asked to further extend his great toe. Maximal plantar flexion may reproduce foot pain but fails to be pathognomonic for anterior tarsal tunnel syndrome. Electromyographical studies may help differentiate this syndrome from proximal peroneal nerve compression or L5 nerve root lesions.[8]

TREATMENT

Conservative therapy should be used initially to treat anterior tarsal tunnel syndrome. Rest, immobilization of the foot at 90° avoiding compression over the tunnel, physical therapy, anti-inflammatory medication, or local corticosteroid injections may relieve the symptoms. In extreme cases, surgical decompression or even sectioning of the nerve at the tunnel's entrance has been suggested to avoid neuroma formation and tendon fixation.

REFERENCES

1. Marinacci, A. A., *Electromyography,* 8, 123, 1968.
2. Kopell, H. P. and Thompson, W. A. L., *Peripheral Entrapment Neuropathies,* William and Wilkins Co., Baltimore, 1963.
3. Mumenthaler, M. and Schliack, H., *Läsionen peripherer Nerven,* G. Thieme, Stuttgart, 1965.
4. Kravatte, M. A., *J. Am. Podiatr. Assoc.,* 61, 457, 1971.
5. Gessini, I., Janolo, B., and Pietrangeli, A., *J. Bone Joint Surg.,* 66A, 786, 1984.
6. Cangialosi, C. P. and Schnall, S. J., *J. Am. Podiatr. Assoc.,* 70, 291, 1980.
7. Borgese, L. F., Hallett, M., Selkoe, D. J., and Welch, K., *J. Neurosurg.,* 54, 89, 1981.
8. Krause, K. H., Witt, T., and Ross, A., *J. Neurol.,* 217, 67, 1977.

TARSAL TUNNEL SYNDROME

Accompanied by their corresponding arteries and veins, the tibial nerve's two terminal branches, the medial and the lateral plantar nerves, pass around the medial malleolus through a fibro-osseus tunnel, the tarsal tunnel (Figure 1). Compression of the nerve produces a clinical picture which was simultaneously described by Keck[1] and Lam.[2,3] Multiple names exist for this tunnel: canal calcanéen de Richet, canal tibio-astragalo-calcanéen, canalis malleolis, and canalis plantaris. Anatomical studies suggest that the majority of the nerve compression occurs in the medial tarsal tunnel.[4] To simplify the picture with its analogy to the carpal tunnel syndrome, this chapter will discuss compression of the tibial nerve in the tarsal tunnel as tarsal tunnel syndrome.[5,6]

ANATOMY

The fibro-osseus tarsal tunnel has bony walls consisting of a bony sulcus on the medial side of the calcaneus, the posterior talar process, and the medial malleolus (Figure 2). Pećina et al.[5] found on 103 specimens that at the lower margin of the calcaneal sulcus for the flexor hallucis longus tendon exists a long ridge (variable in development) to which are attached the deep layer of fibers for the abductor hallucis arch. The nerve's sulcus in the calcaneus may vary from shallow (8 to 10 mm, 23%) or medium (11 to 13 mm, 64%) to deep (14 to 16 mm, 13%).[5] Nerves running in a shallow sulcus are possibly more susceptible to compression. The medial wall of the tunnel is formed by the ligamentum lacinatum and tendinous arch of the abductor hallucis muscle. Tendons overlie this fibro-osseus vault. The ligamentum lacinatum has two layers, a deep and a superficial layer. The superficial layer is a thickening of the crural fascia between the medial malleolus and the calcaneal tuberosity. The deep layer originates from the medial malleolus and passes over the sustentaculum tali and posterior talar process to insert in the crural fascia. The deep layer divides the tunnel into two lacunae: a tendinous lacuna for the tendons of the posterior tibial, the flexor digitorum longus, and the flexor hallucis longus muscles and a neurovascular lacuna.[7]

Lying below the ligamentum lacinatum, the tendinous arch of the abductor hallucis muscle also consists of a superficial and a deep fibrous layer. The superficial layer originates from the calcaneal tuberosity, crosses over the calcaneal sulcus, and reaches the medial malleolus. The deep layer follows the same course to the middle of the tunnel before branching to reach the bony ridge of the calcaneus.[5] When an individual is erect, the deep layer divides the neurovascular structures into an upper and a lower section, (Figure 3), which respectively supply the medial and the lateral plantar areas via their respective plantar sulcus. Just as the posterior tibial artery in the neurovascular lacuna divides into a lateral and a medial plantar artery both of which are accompanied by their corresponding veins, the tibial nerve divides into a medial and a lateral plantar nerve which accompany their vascular supply separated by only a thin membrane. The tarsal tunnel can be considered the hilum of the plantar surface, since virtually all of its neurovascular supply enters through it. These divisions within the tarsal tunnel allow Heimkes et al.[8] to describe a proximal and a distal syndrome.

Before entering the tarsal tunnel, the tibial nerve sends a calcaneus branch to supply the heel's skin. This nerve may be compressed at the edge of the lacinate ligament and lead to the heel pain of calcaneal nerve entrapment.[9] However, not all heel pain can be considered calcaneal nerve entrapment. Compression of the lateral plantar nerve as it passes below the heel to supply the abductor digiti quinti muscle also produces heel pain.

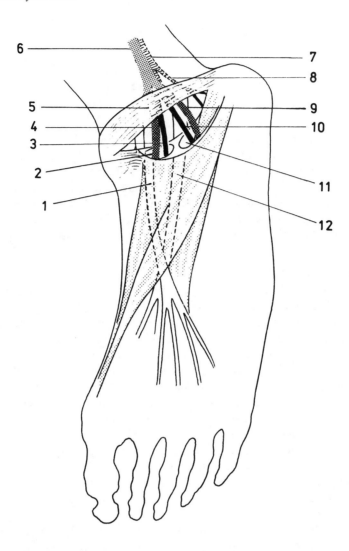

FIGURE 1.   This figure reveals the complex anatomy the tarsal tunnel.
1: Flexor digitorum muscle; 2: upper (medial) tarsal tunnel; 3: medial plantar
nerve; 4: medial plantar artery; 5 ligamentum lacinaatum; 6: posterior tibial
artery; 7: tibial nerve; 8: calcaaneal branches of the tibial nerve; 9: lateral plantar
artery; 10: lateral plantar nerve; 11: lower (lateral) tarsal tunnel; 12: flexor
hallucis longus muscle.

Investigations by Pećina et al.[5] reveal that the upper section of the tarsal tunnel is narrower than the lower section. Therefore, the medial plantar neurovascular structures are not only closer to the tendinous lacuna but also are in a narrower tunnel than the lateral plantar vessels. These anatomical facts place the medial plantar vessels in the medial tarsal tunnel at higher risk for compression. The plantar neurovascular distribution can be seen in Figure 4.

ETIOLOGY

While having nerve compression or irritation in common, the etiologies for tarsal tunnel syndrome are quite diverse, as shown in Table 1. Mechanical pressure from changes in the tissue relationships within the tunnel remains the common denominator of the proposed etiologies. Therefore, trauma and congenital or acquired anomalies predispose these individuals to a higher

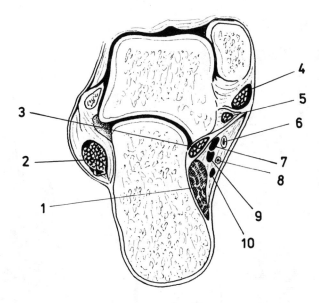

FIGURE 2.   This figure provides a cross section of the tarsal tunnel.
1: Abductor hallucis muscle; 2: peroneus longus muscle; 3: flexor
hallucis longus muscle; 4: posterior tibial muscle; 5: flexor digitorum
longus muscle; 6: medial plantar artery; 7: medial plantar nerve; 8:
lateral plantar artery; 9: lateral plantar nerve; 10: calcaneal branches of
the tibial nerve.

risk of nerve compression, since their tarsal tunnel is abnormal in configuration. Rather than changing the bony components, autoimmune and inflammatory diseases affect the tunnel's soft tissues and decrease the tunnel's volume.[10-13] Since the tunnel's neural components remain most sensitive to increased pressure, changes in sensory and motor function are among the first symptoms of tunnel damage.[14,15] The upper section of the tunnel containing the medial plantar neurovascular structures remains more sensitive to volume changes than the lower section containing the lateral plantar neurovascular structures.

The tibial nerve, like the median nerve, has a rich vascularity but is sensitive to ischemia. Compression of the vasa vasorum surrounding the nerve will lead to ischemia and neurological symptoms.[16-18] Increased vascular compromise during standing and walking account for the crises appreciated in patients with tarsal tunnel syndrome. In several idiopathic cases that have been relieved after surgery, the nerves were found to be normal in appearance. These cases have been proposed to be vascular in nature. However, idiopathic cases remain as such until their causes become clarified.

CLINICAL SYMPTOMS AND SIGNS

The clinical picture of tarsal tunnel syndrome is characterized by pain and paresthesia, especially in the dermatome of the medial plantar nerve, the medial plantar surface, and the great, second, and third toes (Figure 4). Predominantly affecting the toes, the pain is accompanied by burning, numbness, pressure, or feelings of pins and needles. These symptoms become crises when they worsen at night or after long periods of standing or walking. Proximal irradiation of pain can lead to an erroneous diagnosis of sciatica, lumbosacral spine disease, or proximal neurological compromise. Patients may even present with bilateral tarsal tunnel syndrome.[19]

Objective signs can be difficult to detect. While anesthesia or hyperesthesia is rare, hypesthesia and loss of two-point discrimination are early signs of nerve compression. Tinel's sign, one of the more constant objective findings, can usually be provoked in tarsal tunnel

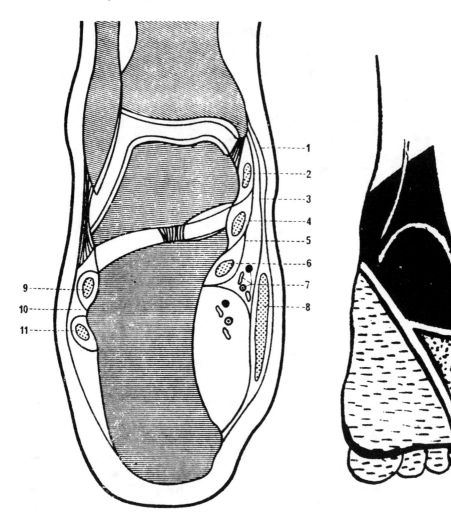

FIGURE 3.   This figure shows a cross section of the tunnel with attention to the relationships of the upper tarsal tunnel.
1: Ligamentum lacinatum; 2: posterior tibial muscle; 3: tendinous arch of the abductor hallucis muscle; 4: flexor digitorum longus muscle; 5: deep layer of the ligamentum lacinatum; 6: flexor hallucis longus muscle; 7: the neurovascular bundle in the upper tarsal tunnel; 8: abductor hallucis muscle; 9: peroneus brevis muscle; 10: canal of the peroneal muscles; 11: peroneus longus muscle.

FIGURE 4.   This schematic delineates the dermatomes of the nerves passing through the tarsal tunnel: the calcaneal branches (black), the medial plantar nerve (hatched), and the later plantar nerve (dotted).

syndrome. Sometimes sweating may be reduced. Inspection of the ankle may reveal a retromalleolar or submalleolar swelling. Forced eversion (pronation) and dorsi-flexion of the foot can reproduce pain and paresthesia in the nerve's distribution.[20] Abduction of the toes may also cause pain. While occasionally felt throughout the plantar surface, the symptoms are usually confined to the dermatome of the medial plantar nerve. This indicates compression of the upper section of the tunnel. However, to avoid confusion between complete and partial tarsal tunnel syndrome, both presentations will be considered tarsal tunnel syndrome.

Muscular dysfunction may be hard to detect by a superficial examination. Since the long flexors of the foot and toes are preserved, patients have no difficulty standing or walking. While the effects of carpal tunnel syndrome on one's hands are well noticed, the effects of tibial nerve compression may go unnoticed since the foot is not typically used for precise movements.

TABLE 1
**Proposed Etiologies of Tarsal Tunnel Syndrome by Their Action and
General Category.**

Category	Action	Specific etiology
Trauma	Change in anatomical	Exostoses (Carayon and Courbil, 1965[28]); medial malleolar fracture;talus fracture — posterior process; dislocation of the ankle; joint changes (Kenzora et al., 1982[29]); post-traumatic arthritis (Komar and Banky, 1966;[30] Mosimann and Mumenthaler, 1969[31]); i.v. infusions and scarring in the saphenous vein (Serre et al., 1965[12]); shallow sulcus (Pećina et al., 1968[5]); anomalies of the ankle (vertical talus) valgus deformity/varus heels/pronated splayed forefeet (Radin, 1983[32])
Congenital/ acquired	Initial tunnel configuration	Malformation of posterior process talus (Mosimann and Mumenthaler, 1969[31]); hypertrophy of abductor hallucis muscle (Edwards et al., 1969[27])
Autoimmune	Connective tissue disease, spartial relationship	Rheumatoid arthritis (McGuigan et al., 1983[33]); amyloid; sarcoidosis; dermatomyositis; gout; scleroderma; systemic disease (Oloff et al., 1983[13])
Inflammatory tenosynovitis/	Space in the tunnel	Ankylosing spondylitis (Enright et al., 1979[34]); tendonitis (Kenzora et al., 1982[29])
Metabolic/ hormonal	Tissue effects	Diabetes; pregnancy; myxoedema; acromegaly osteoporosis (Byrd, 1981[35]); hyperlipidemia (Ruderman et al., 1983[36])
Tumors	Space-occupying lesions	Ganglion (Matricali, 1980;[37] Brown, 1982[38]); lipoma, neurilemoma (Dowling and Skaggs, 1982[39]); cysts, neurofibroma (Marinacci, 1957, 1968[40,41])
Vascular	Space in tunnel	Varicose veins (Gould and Alvarez, 1983;[42] Pećina, 1987[43]); venous plexus (Keck, 1962[1]); peripheral occlusive disease (Greiter and Wilde, 1970[44]) stasis secondary to occupations requiring long periods of standing; ischemic changes in nerve
Idiopathic		Lam, 1962;[2] Keck, 1962;[1] McGill, 1964;[45] Kopell and Thompson, 1960;[46] Marinacci 1957;[40] Bora and Ostermann, 1982[47]

The clinical picture does not include primary vascular signs, since the vascular structures are more resistant to compression. However, several vascular disorders have been postulated to lead to neural compromise.

Diagnosis of tarsal tunnel syndrome requires a full evaluation, including radiographic and electromyographic studies. Axial radiographs of the calcaneous reveal the bony structure of the tunnel (Figure 5). In early, confusing cases, electrodiagnostic studies may be of considerable value in evaluation, progression of compression, and nerve recovery.[21] Kaplan and Kernahan,[22] emphasize the importance of decreased amplitude and increased duration of evoked potentials rather than distal motor latency. Oh et al.[23] use these studies to rule out S1 root compression from the differential diagnosis. Negative electromyographic and normal conduction velocity studies do not exclude the possibility of tarsal tunnel syndrome.[20,24,25] A vascular evaluation in nondiabetic patients will clarify the vascular supply to the lower extremity. The differential diagnosis includes arch problems, Morton's metatarsalgia, lumbosacral spine disorders (i.e., bony disorder, spurs), calcaneodynia, and plantar fasciitis.

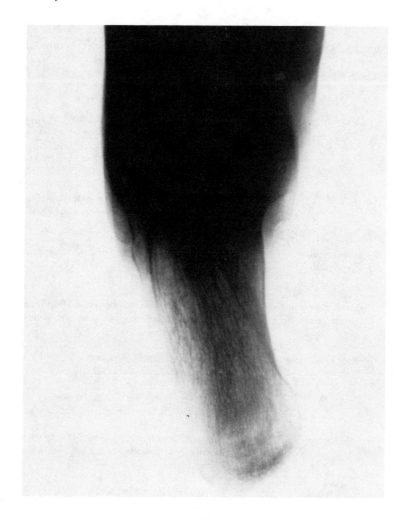

FIGURE 5.   The components of the tarsal tunnel run along the calcaneus and are bound to the bone by the ligaments and tendons accompanying the nerves into the foot. Bony abnormalities can deform the tunnel and lead to nerve compression.

TREATMENT

Conservative therapy removes the causes of compression and treats the primary disease (Figure 6). Rest, avoidance of repetitive trauma, immobilization (plaster casts), use of orthotics, physical therapy, anti-inflammatory medication, and local corticosteroid injection may be tried in several combinations to yield success rates up to 79% (19/24) as shown by Androić.[26]

Surgical therapy should be initiated if the symptoms have persisted 6 months, conservative therapy has failed to being relief, or muscle atrophy exists. While not without risk, one may repeat corticosteroid injections up to three times within 2 months before considering surgery.

Operative treatment can relieve the compression by releasing the ligamentous bands, removing the offending agents (i.e., inflamed synovium, ganglions, exostoses, osteophytes), and occasionally performing a neurolysis. Sectioning of the superficial layer of the lacinate ligament is not sufficient The deep layer must be sectioned but preserved, since it is important not only as an origin for the abductor hallucis muscle, but also as a foot stabilizer. Following surgical release, patients should be immobilized up to 2 weeks before starting motion. Operative results can be as excellent as 88% (14/16), as described by Edwards et al.[27]

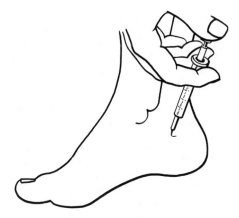

FIGURE 6.   Conservative therapy for tarsal tunnel may include the injection of corticosteroid into the tunnel.

REFERENCES

1. Keck, Ch., *J. Bone Joint Surg.,* 44A, 180, 1962.
2. Lam, S. J. S., *Lancet,* 2, 1354, 1962.
3. Lam. S. J. S., *J. Bone Joint Surg.,* 49B, 87, 1967.
4. Komar, J., *Alagut-szindromak,* Medicina Könyvkiado, Budapest, 1977.
5. Pećina, M., Zergollern, J., and Novoselac, M., *Lijec. Vjesn.,* 90, 23, 1968.
6. Zergollern, J. and Pecina, M., *Reumatizam,* 14, 208, 1967.
7. Kiljman, J., *Acta Chir. Lugosl.,* 1, 40, 1954.
8. Heimkes, B., Posel, P., Stotz, S., and Wolf, K., *Int. Orthop.,* 11, 193, 1987.
9. Deese, M. J. and Baxter, E. D., *J. Musculoskeletal Med.,* 68, 1988.
10. Denis, M. A., *Rev. Rhum. Mal. Osteoartic.,* 32, 106, 1965.
11. Robecchi, A., *Reumatismo,* 17, 319, 1965.
12. Serre, H., Simon, L., Claustre, J., and Avile de Azevede, M., *Rev. Rhum. Mal. Ostcoartic.,* 32, 96, 1965.
13. Oloff, L. M., Jacobs, A. M., and Jaffe, S., *J. Foot Surg.,* 22, 302, 1983.
14. Sidey, J. D., *Lancet,* 1, 496, 1963.
15. Kravatte, M. A., *J. Am. Podiatr. Assoc.,* 61, 457, 1971.
16. Fullerton, P. M., *J. Neurol. Neurosurg. Psychiatr.,* 26, 385, 1963.
17. Galinski, A. W., *J. Am. Podiatr. Assoc.,* 60, 169, 1970.
18. Pećina, M., Zbornik radova IV simpozija o bolestima i ozljedama sake, Opatija, 1974, str. 203.
19. Goodman, C. R. and Kehr, L. E., *J. Am. Podiatr. Assoc.,* 73, 256, 1983.
20. Mumenthaler, M., Probst, Ch., Mumenthaler, A., Weber, B. G., and Schyder, J., *Schweiz. Med. Wochenschr.,* 94, 373, 1964.
21. Goodgold, J., Kopell, H. P., and Spielholz, N. J., *N. Engl. J. Med.,* 267, 742, 1965.
22. Kaplan, E. and Kernahan, T., *J. Bone Joint Surg.,* 63A, 96, 1981.
23. Oh, S. J., Sarala, P. K., Kuba, T., and Elmore, R. S., *Ann. Neurol.,* 5, 327, 1978.
24. Gathier, J. C., Gruyn, G. W., and van der Meer, W. K., *Psychiatr. Neurol. Neurochir.,* 73, 97, 1970.
25. Séze, S., Dreyfus, P., Denis, A., et al., *Ann. Med. Phys.,* 13, 133, 1970.
26. Androić, S., *Reumatizam,* 14, 12, 1967.
26a. Androić, S., *Reumatizam,* 18, 95, 1971.
27. Edwards, W. G., Lincoln, C. R., Basset, F. H., and Goldner, J. L., *JAMA,* 207, 716, 1969.
28. Carayon, A. and Courbil, J. L., *Ann. Chir.,* 19, 1538, 1965.
29. Kenzora, J. E., Lenet, M. D., and Sherman, M., *Foot Ankle,* 3, 181, 1982.
30. Komar, J. and Banky, F., *Munch. Med. Wochenschr.,* 708, 1115, 1966.
31. Mosimann, W. and Mumenthaler, M., *Helv. Chir. Acta,* 36, 547, 1969.
32. Radin, E. L., *Clin. Orthop.,* 181, 167, 1983.

33. McGuigan, L., Burke, D., and Fleming, A., *Ann. Rheum. Dis.,* 42, 128, 1983.
34. Enright, T., Liang, G. C., Fox, T. A., and Mueller, R. F., *Arthritis Rheum.,* 22, 77, 1979.
35. Byrd, J. W., Ricciardi, J. M., and Jung, B. I., *Clin. Orthop.,* 157, 164, 1981.
36. Ruderman, M. I., Palmer, R. H., Oiaste, M. R., Lovelace, R. E., Haas, R., Rowland, L. P., *Arch. Neurol.,* 40, 124, 1983.
37. Matricali, B., *J. Neurosurg.,* 24, 183, 1980.
38. Brown, R. J., *Ulster Med. J.,* 51, 127, 1982.
39. Dowling, G. L. and Skaggs, R. E., *J. Am. Podiatr. Assoc.,* 72, 45, 1982.
40. Marinacci, A. A., *Bull. L. A. Neurol. Soc.,* 22, 171, 1957.
41. Marinacci, A. A., *Bull. L. A. Neurol. Soc.,* 33, 90, 1968.
42. Gould, N. and Alvarez, R., *Foot Ankle,* 3, 290, 1983.
43. Pećina, M. and Krmpotic-Nemanic, J., Kanalikularni Sindromi, Med. fak., Zagreb, 1987.
44. Greiter, Th. E. and Wilde, A. H., *Cleve. Clin. Q.,* 37, 23, 1970.
45. McGill, D. A., Proc. R. Soc. Med., 57, 1125, 1964.
46. Kopell, H. P. and Thompson, W. A. L., *N. Engl. J. Med.,* 262, 56, 1960.
47. Bora, F. W. and Ostermann, A. L., *Clin. Orthop.,* 163, 20, 1982.

METATARSALGIA

Metatarsalgia has become a common name for multiple disorders arising from pain in the forefoot. Debating the true meaning of metatarsalgia goes beyond the scope of this chapter; however, compression of nerves in the metatarsal tunnels produces forefoot pain commonly known as Morton's neuroma, Morton's metatarsalgia, neuroma plantaris, or Morton's disease.

ANATOMY

The metatarsal tunnels lie between the superficial and deep transverse metatarsal ligaments (ligamentum metatarseum transversum profundum and superficiale), which connect the metatarsal heads. The medial and lateral plantar nerves and the medial and lateral plantar arteries and veins produce the common digital neurovascular bundle that transverses the metatarsal tunnels. The medial and the lateral plantar nerves supply branches to the first, second, and third metatarsal spaces, and the third and fourth metatarsal spaces, respectively. These fields on the plantar surface have minimal overlap. The medial plantar nerve also supplies the great toe, while the lateral plantar nerve supplies the fifth toe. The branch to the great toe originates as the medial plantar nerve leaves the tarsal tunnel. The common digital branches from the medial plantar nerves originate at a branch point over the first and second metatarsal bases. Anesthesic injection into this area distal to the medial cuneiform bone will produce complete anesthesia of the first and second metatarsal spaces, since the third space receives some innervation from the lateral plantar nerve. Within the tunnels, the common digital nerves branch into the digitales proprii nerves for the medial and lateral plantar skin of the corresponding toes (ie., the first metatarsal space lies between the great and second toe; thus, there is a lateral branch to the great toe and a medial branch to the second toe). The tendons of the flexor muscles and the interossei muscles contribute to the tunnel formed by the transverse ligaments and the metatarsal heads.

ETIOLOGY

While the pathology was first described by Durlacher in 1894,[1] Thomas Morton[2] in 1876 first postulated compressive neuropathy as the etiology. Tubby provided operative data detailing a neuroma-like swelling between the metatarsal heads.[3] Prolonged compression and irritation of the neurovascular bundle leads to endoneural edema, nerve fiber degeneration with reparative changes and thickening of the nerve, and hyaline changes and thickening of the vessel's walls.[4] Multiple authors have described the etiology as that of an entrapment neuropathy.[5-9]

While many etiologies have been proposed, most require a change in the metatarsal tunnel size. Trauma, inflammatory diseases, functional anatomy, and degenerative changes of the tunnel's tissues probably provide the changes necessary to compress or to irritate the nerve.[10-13] Hormonal factors producing edema, which can be found in pregnant or premenstrual women,[14,15] and nerve ischemia[16] have also been presented as etiologies. However, the interdependence of all of these factors makes it statistically difficult to isolate the basic causes. Since the neurovascular structures are nearly at their terminal point, local nerve ischemia can easily result from compression.

In the development of metatarsalgia, distortion of the metatarsophalangeal joints from trauma plays a major role. Fractures or subluxation of the joint change the anatomy of the tunnel. Osteochondritis of the second metatarsal head (Morbus Kohler-Frieberg) can lead to tunnel narrowing.[17] Minimal variation in the tunnel anatomy may lead to metatarsalgia if only repetitive nerve irritation from the anterior margin of the transverse metatarsal ligament is needed.[18] Other causes of compression include rheumatic inflammatory diseases, ganglions, and synovial cysts.[19]

The anatomical relationships of the metatarsal tunnel have been proposed as the basic uniting theory.[5,20] Since all of the above etiologies affect the static and, therefore, the dynamic anatomy of the metatarsal tunnel, simple anatomical relationships cannot be the sole cause of metatarsalgia. However, foot motion and position alter the anatomy of the tunnel. Distortion and variation in the relationships of the metatarsal heads will affect the size of the tunnel. Congenital and acquired abnormalities of the entire leg may affect the weight-bearing status of the foot, predisposing to nerve compression in the region of the metatarsal heads. Due most frequently to shoes with high heels or narrow toe boxes,[21] hyperextension of the toes narrows the metatarsal tunnels. Crouching duplicates the position found with high-heeled shoes; therefore, men whose professions require long periods of crouching may present with metatarsalgia. Flexion contractures of the hip and knee, pes equinus, digiti mallei, and other foot deformations also lead to toe hyperextension to compensate for the more proximal abnormalities.

CLINICAL SYMPTOMS AND SIGNS

In 1876, Thomas Morton[2] described metatarsalgia as follows: "In walking paroxismal pain appears, pain that goes to the heart and provokes unbearable sensations with cold sweat and finally prevents the individual to direct his spirit and will to any other subject but to this unbearable pain." This picture remains accurate today. Pain appears cutting or electrical in sensation but never diffuse and burning, like plantar fasciitis. Toe hyperextension in high-heeled shoes or while crouching aggravates the pain. Patients will even describe having to stop their work and remove their shoes. Avoiding shoes with high heels or narrow toe boxes may eliminate the pain. However, trouble may persist regardless of an individual's footwear.

Clinical examination reveals a trigger point at the metatarsal heads, especially between the third and fourth heads (the third metatarsal space). The second and fourth metatarsal spaces are less frequently involved, and the first metatarsal space is rarely involved. Compression of the metatarsal heads against each other provokes and increases the pain. While typically masked by the pain, hypoanalgesia or analgesia on the skin of the involved toes may be appreciated. Morton's metatarsalgia should not be confused either by name nor clinical findings with Morton's foot (Neanderthal foot, short first metatarsal bone), when the worst pain localizes to the basis of the first and second metatarsal bones.[22] In an attempt to improve the accuracy of diagnosis, Guiloff et al.[9] conducted clinical and electrophysiological examinations of 16 patients with atypical foot pain. Guiloff et al.[9] concluded that nerve conduction velocity studies were helpful in clarifying the diagnosis.

TREATMENT

Removal of the provocative causes may be accomplished by several approaches. The conservative approaches try to avoid high-heeled shoes and shoes with narrow toe boxes, to keep the foot from prolonged plantar flexion or toe extension, and to support the metatarsal heads with a pad proximal to the heads, with simultaneous support of the longitudinal foot arch. Physical therapies, anti-inflammatory medication, and local injection of corticosteroid and anesthetic have been found to be effective (Figures 1 and 2).[23,24] Rather than inject the tunnel with additional fluid, Krmpotić-Nemanić et al.[23,24] recommended injection distal to the leading edge of the medial cuneifrom bone, as shown in Figure 3. While the needle may come close to the medial plantar nerve and produce pain through its distribution, the corticosteroid injection should be placed around the nerve. The local anesthetic included will provide sudden but temporary disappearance of the symptoms and temporary anesthesia in the nerve's dermatome. If removal of aggravating factors is continued, the use of local corticosteroid injection may be repeated to achieve a success rate of 70%. Krmpotić-Nemanić et al.[23,24] found a 70% success rate in the women treated with between three and ten local injections. The remainder required surgical removal of the offending neuroma[6] or, if no neuroma was appreciated, sectioning of the transverse metatarsal ligament. Johnson et al. described the results of reoperation because of persistent pain after excision of an interdigital neuroma.[25]

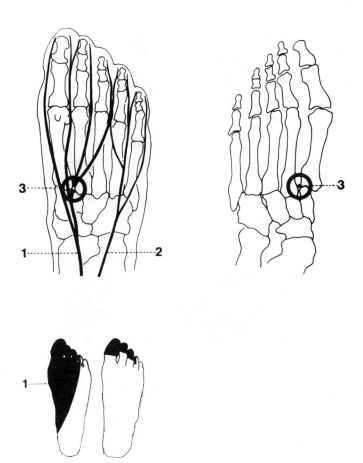

FIGURE 1.   This figure traces the course of the medial (1) and lateral (2) plantar nerves. A diagnostic intervention may include the injection of anesthetic into the space indicated (3). The dermatome of the medial plantar nerve is typically involved and is highlighted on the plantar and dorsal views of the foot

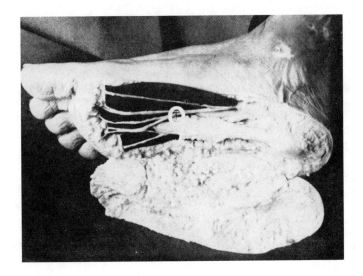

FIGURE 2.   This pathologic specimen has been disected to show the nerve branch point that is injected when a needle is placed in the interspace between the first and second metatarsal bones.

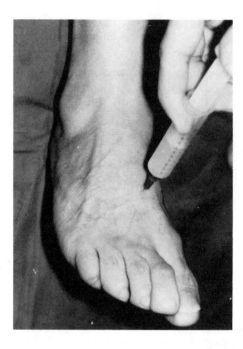

FIGURE 3.   This photograph demonstrates the actual
location of the injection on the dorsum of the foot.

REFERENCES

1. Durlacher, L., A treatise on corns, bunions, the disease of nails, and the general management of the feet, Simpkin Marshall Co., London, 1845.
2. Morton, T. G., *Am. J. Med. Sci.,* 71, 37, 1876.
3. Tubby, A. H., Deformities Including Disease of the Bones and Joints, Mc Millan Co., London, 1912.
4. Lassmann, G. and Machacek, J., *Wien Klin. Wochenschr.,* 81, 55, 1969.
5. Kopell, H. P., and Thompson W. A. L., *Peripheral Entrapment Neuropathies,* Williams and Wilkins, Baltimore, 1963.
6. Lassmann, G., Lassmann, H., and Stockinger, L., *Virchows Arch [A],* 370, 307, 1976.
7. Ochoa, J., *J. Neuropathol. Exp. Neurol.,* 35, 370, 1976.
8. Gauthier, G., *Clin. Orthop.,* 142, 90, 1979.
9. Guiloff, J. R., Scadding, W. J., and Klenerman, L., *J. Bone Joint Surg.,* 66B, 586, 1984.
10. Denis, A., *Actual Rhum.,* 7, 168, 1970.
11. Viladot, A., *Orthop. Clin. North Am.,* 4, 165, 1973.
12. Denis, A., Erkrankungen des Fusses, Fol. rheumat., Ciba-Geigy, Basle, 1974.
13. Bickel, W. H. and Dockerty, M. B., *Surg. Gynecol. Obst.,* 84, 111, 1974.
14. Gospodinoff, A. and Gospodinoff, L., *Policlinico (Sez. Med.) Roma,* 70, 249, 1963.
15. Brown, M. and Lane, M., *Med. J. Aust.,* 1, 929, 1965.
16. Nissen, K. I., *J. Bone Joint Surg.,* 30B, 84, 1948.
17. Du Vries, H. L., *Surgery of the Foot,* C. V. Mosby, St. Louis, 1965.
18. McElvenny, R. T., *J. Bone Joint Surg.,* 25, 675, 1943.
19. Lassmann, G., *Dtsch. Z. Nervenheilk,* 192, 338, 1968.
20. Kravette, M. A., *J. Am. Podiatr. Assoc.,* 61, 457, 1971.
21. Morris, M. A., *Clin. Orthop.,* 127, 203, 1977.
22. Morton, D. J., *The Human Foot,* Columbia University Press, New York, 1948.
23. Krmpotic-Nemanic, J., Keros, P., Pecina, M., Stern-Padovan, R., Vidovic, M., Folia Anat. Lugosl., 5, 7, 1976.
24. Krmpotic-Nemanic, J., Pecina, M., and Kerons, P., *Chir. del Piede,* 4, 57, 1980.
25. Johnson, J. E., Johnson, K. A., and Krishnan Unni, K., *J. Bone Joint Surg.,* 70A, 651, 1988.

Part III

TUNNEL SYNDROMES IN ATHLETES*

In describing individual tunnel syndromes in the upper and lower extremities in the introduction, acute trauma and especially long-term repetitive microtrauma in areas of specific tunnels have been indicated as instigating agents. Certain sports or physical activities have been mentioned that lead to specific tunnel syndromes, for example, cyclist's palsy and bowler's thumb.

Contrary to tunnel syndromes, vascular and neurovascular syndromes in athletes seem to be more familiar and have been much more described, while tunnel syndromes in athletes have been reported only recently. This chapter provides some information about tunnel syndromes in specific athletic activities, with specific reference to each individual tunnel syndrome presented in this book.

Thoracic outlet syndrome includes the three following syndromes: anterior scalene muscle syndrome, costoclavicular syndrome, and hyperabduction syndrome. Although these have been analyzed separately in this book, our aim is to discuss them under the common name of neurovascular obstruction, which has already been described in sports, especially with regard to swimming and other activities within which swing motion of the arm is required (e.g., throwing).[1-3] Compression of neurovascular structures through the costoclavicular space is usually caused by dynamic changes, especially in shoulder girdle mechanics, i.e., functional anatomy of the shoulder girdle. The scapula is actually suspended by muscles. Injuries such as direct blows, sudden traction, or long-term repetitive strains leads to shoulder depression, which results in the narrowing of costoclavicular space, thereby causing clinical symptoms of the thoracic outlet syndrome. In the most recent literature the insidious onset of the shoulder girdle depression without any known outer causes has been discussed.[4] The idea is that tennis players and pitchers develop shoulder-girdle depression due to multiple factors: greater muscular mass of the dominant limb and repetitive microtrauma causing stretching of the scapula suspensory and stabilizing musculature.[2] Therefore, it is recommended for athletes with neurovascular symptoms in the upper extremity to pay attention to postural abnormalities or the existence of *scapula suspensory insufficiency*. The coracoid process and the pectoralis minor muscle insertion act as a fulcrum over which the neurovascular structures change direction when the arm is elevated. This site has been implicated as a source of neurovascular compression among athletes who repetitively hyperabduct the arm — swimmers, tennis players, pitchers.[1] In swimmers, neurovascular compression in this area may develop as a result of the pectoralis minor muscle hypertrophy.[5] The most frequent symptoms of thoracic outlet syndrome are related to compression of the lower trunk of the brachial plexus and, to a lesser degree, to compression of the upper trunk of the brachial plexus. When the site of pain is in the shoulder girdle, neck, or face, a C5-C6 disc herniation must be considered in the differential diagnosis. Vascular symptoms are quite rare, and a clinical distinction may be made between venous compression, whose symptoms include arm edema, cyanosis, and venous collateralization across the shoulder and chest wall, and arterial compression, whose symptoms include coolness, numbness, and exertional fatigue. A final symptom pattern in thoracic outlet syndrome is that of *mixed involvement*. However, the dominant character of the compression may vary from a top basketball player, in whom arterial compression symptoms have been observed, to a top water polo pivotman whose only symptoms were of venous compression. Both athletes were initially treated nonoperatively, including correction of postural abnormalities and an exercise program for strengthening the scapular suspensory muscles. Both athletes abstained from intensive exercises and were not able to participate in half of their competitive season. However upon

* Written by Ivan Bojanić, M.D., Marko Pećina, M.D. Ph.D., and Andrew D. Markiewitz, M.D.

rehabilitation, they successfully returned to their teams and played regularly at a competitive level. Nevertheless, in certain cases where an explicit anatomical abnormality leads to compression, surgical decompression is indicated. Surgery is indicated in athletes with dynamic neurovascular compression when nonoperative treatment or conservative therapy does not relieve their symptoms. A first-rib resection through a transaxillary approach is recommended, and in most of the cases excellent results have been accomplished.[2,3]

Backpack paralysis, though not mentioned in the section on thoracic outlet syndrome bears mention here because it is actually compression of the brachial plexus. Compression of the brachial plexus may arise from both intrinsic and extrinsic factors. Both of these mechanisms may occur in association with athletic endeavor. The most common external agent creating compression of the brachial plexus is a knapsack.[6-8] In Hirasawa and Sakakida's series,[7] most of the observed brachial plexus lesions were described as "backpack paralysis." Brachial plexus compression results when large, heavy backpacks are carried for long periods. The shoulder girdle is pulled posteriorly by the heavy pack, adding a component of traction. Treatment of backpack paralysis combines avoiding the mechanisms thought to have caused it and participating in physical therapy. Physical therapy restores one's strength, allowing complete recovery.

Traumatic injury of the axillary nerve is commonly seen in athletes. It occurs most commonly as a result of an acute anterior shoulder dislocation. Blunt trauma to the shoulder occurring during football or wrestling has also been implicated as a possible cause of nerve injury.[9] Entrapment of the axillary nerve in the quadrilateral space is rare in athletes. It has been described in baseball pitchers.[10]

Suprascapular nerve entrapment is an infrequently observed disorder and is often misdiagnosed. The manner of presentation of this syndrome depends on the anatomical site of neurologic compression. Entrapment usually occur at the suprascapular notch. Patients, mostly throwing athletes, present with poorly localized shoulder pain, intact sensation, weakness of external rotation and abduction, and atrophy of the supraspinatus and the infraspinatus muscle.[11-13] Occasionally entrapment occur distally, at the spinoglenoid notch. Patients may be asymptomatic or may describe mild pain and weakness of the shoulder because of denervation of the infraspinatus.[14-16] Ferretti et al.[14] found 12 top-level volleyball players with an isolated asymptomatic paralysis of the infraspinatus muscle. Ganzhorn et al.[17] described the case of a weight lifter who presented after noting wasting in the region of dorsal scapula while posing in the mirror.

Radial nerve nontraumatic compression above the elbow is rare in athletes. It has been reported following strenuous muscular activities that require repeated elbow extension against resistance, such as weight lifting.[18] The site of compression is in the region of the lateral intermuscular septum, which the radial nerve pierces as it enters the anterior aspect of the arm, 10 cm proximal to the lateral epicondyle.[19]

Posterior interosseous nerve entrapment results in a purely motor deficit with no sensory complaints and no loss of sensation. It is described in throwing sports, skiing, and those activities that demand repetitive, tight grips, such as golf, tennis, and weight lifting.[20] The literature indicates that the posterior interosseous nerve syndrome coexists in 5% of those with lateral epicondylitis (tennis elbow).[21]

In their study of a group of patients with chronic tennis elbow, Roles and Maudsley[22] recognized the radial nerve within its tunnel and called it **"radial tunnel syndrome."** The syndrome differs from a posterior interosseous nerve syndrome, in which the problem is localized to compression of the nerve at one particular site, the arcade of Frohse, and results in only a motor deficit. In a radial tunnel syndrome, there may be a spectrum of complaints, including pain, paresthesias, and weakness. A motor deficit is not nearly as common as in a posterior interosseous syndrome.[23] There are five potential sites of compression within the radial tunnel: fibrous bands at its proximal portion, a fibrous medial edge along the extensor carpi radialis brevis, a "fan" of radial recurrent vessels, the arcade of Fröhse, and lastly, a fibrous band at the distal edge of the supinator muscle. The radial tunnel syndrome occurs most commonly in tennis players, but may also be seen in rowers and weight lifters.[18,24] Nonoperative measures should be the first form of treatment. Such measures include rest of the elbow and wrist from repetitive stressful activity and a course of anti-inflammatory medication. Surgical exploration with neurolysis is indicated if nonoperative treatment fails. Several authors have reported good and excellent results in a high percentage of patients.[25,26]

Athletes involved in sports requiring repetitive pronation supination ulnar flexion activities may acquire **Wartenberg's disease — entrapment of the superficial sensory branch of the radial nerve** in the forearm.[27] Wearing of wrist bands as in racquet sports has also been implicated as a cause of this syndrome, also known as handcuff neuropathy.[20,27-29]

Ulnar nerve entrapment at the elbow is most frequently encountered in the throwing athletes, such as in baseball pitchers, tennis players, and javelin throwers, but is also observed in skiing, weight lifting, and stick-handling sports.[8,30-33] Because of its position in the cubital tunnel, the ulnar nerve is vulnerable to repetitive tension or traction stresses in athletes. This may also be compounded by subluxation or instability of the nerve. Childress[34] reported that 16.2% of the population demonstrated recurrent dislocation of the ulnar nerve when the elbow was flexed and extended. Repeated stress and injury may lead to inflammation, adhesions, and a progressive compressive neuropathy. The intermittent nature of the athletic endeavors may confuse the presentation of the athlete with entrapment of the ulnar nerve at the elbow. Sometimes the first presenting symptom will consist of pain along the medial joint line that is either associated with or exacerbated by overhead activities. As the inflammation of the nerve progresses, pain and paresthesias will be noted down the ulnar aspect of the forearm to the hand. Sensory changes definitely precede motor changes; however, a careful evaluation of the interingic musculature of the hand is essential to detect any weakness. Quite often, recalcitrant ulnar nerve entrapment at the elbow requires surgery. However, many transient episodes can be treated nonoperatively. Del Pizzo et al.[30] reported 19 baseball players who underwent surgery for ulnar nerve entrapment at the elbow. The surgery consisted of anterior transfer of the nerve deep to the origin of the flexor muscles. Of 15 players followed up, 9 had returned to baseball.

Entrapment of the ulnar nerve in Guyon's canal (ulnar tunnel yndrome) is seen in cyclists and racquetball players as a result of chronic external compression. The first report of ulnar neuropathy as a complication of long-distance cycling was published in 1896.[35] Several reports have since described this complication, called cyclist's or handlebar palsy.[36-40] Factors reported in the literature as contributing to the development of neuropathies in cyclists include the use of worn-out gloves, unpadded handlebars, prolonged grasping of dropped handlebars, riding an improperly adjusted bicycle, and vibratory trauma from rough roads. Jackson[40] recently studied 20 cyclists with riding experience of more than 100 miles per week and found that 9 of 20 cyclists complained of either hand or finger numbness during cycling that resolved after completion of the ride. They reported that their hand numbness or pain was reduced after adjusting their hand position. Conventional treatment for nerve compression syndrome at the wrist consists of changes in cycling technique, including frequently varying hand position, the use of properly padded gloves and handlebars, and changes in the bicycle that ensure a proper fit. These changes frequently will relieve symptoms, in most cases without need for surgical decompression of the Guyon's canal. Repetitive trauma to the heel of the palm can cause ulnar artery spasms, thromboses, or aneurysms and, thus, compromise the ulnar nerve function with a more vascular type of presentation. This condition, known as hypothenar hammer syndrome, has been described in conjunction with several sports, including karate, judo, tennis, and lacrosse.[27,41,42] Nonunion of the hook of the hamate or of the pisiform, which may be fractured during a tennis, baseball, or golf swing, can also cause entrapment within the ulnar tunnel (Guyon's canal).[20] It is also important to keep in mind the possibility of a double crush injury of the ulnar nerve with coexistence of the syndrome of the flexor carpi ulnaris muscle (cubital tunnel syndrome) and ulnar tunnel syndrome.

Entrapment of the median nerve at the elbow is termed the "pronator teres syndrome" and may result from repetitive exercise and resultant hypertrophy of the flexor-pronator muscle group.[25,43] Patients complain of pain and tenderness in the volar aspect of their forearms over the area of compression that worsens with exertional activities. Sensory complaints are common, consisting of numbness and paresthesias in part or all of the median nerve distribution of the hand. The pronator teres syndrome is often a difficult diagnosis and must be distinguished from carpal tunnel syndrome.

Anterior interosseous syndrome (Kiloh-Nevin syndrome) has been described in association with repetitive activities such as throwing, racquet sports, or weight lifting.[18,44] It is characterized by a vague feeling of discomfort in the proximal forearm that may mimic a pronator teres syndrome. The classic finding is the patient who loses the ability to pinch between his thumb and index finger. However, this is not always present.

The incidence of **carpal tunnel syndrome** as a sport-related problem is surprisingly low. It may be seen in sports secondary to gripping, throwing, cycling, repetitive wrist flexion/extension activity, as well as direct trauma.[7,20,24,25,27,43,45,46] Since carpal tunnel syndrome is so rare in the athlete, unusual causes must be suspected when the diagnosis is entertained.

Digital nerve syndromes in the athlete are less common than syndromes occurring at the wrist level. Digital nerves may be compressed during their course in the distal palm or at the proximal digit level. Bowler's thumb is the most common syndrome involving the digital nerve in the hand in sports.[20,24,27,43,46-51] Repetitive compression of the ulnar digital nerve to the thumb secondary to direct pressure on the nerve from the thumb hole of a bowling ball has been implicated as a cause of bowler's thumb. Incidently, bowler's thumb has been reported in a baseball player.[20] On physical examination the patients have tenderness over the ulnar volar aspect of the metacarpophalangeal joint of the thumb and a positive Tinel's sign in this area with paresthesias radiating to the ulnar aspect of the tip of the thumb. There is no motor involvement; however, grip strength may be somewhat diminished secondary to pain. Bowler's thumb should be treated nonoperatively with rest, cessation of activity, nonsteroidal anti-inflammatory medication, and modification of equipment and technique. In advanced cases, a molded plastic thumb guard is recommended to prevent trauma. Surgical treatment is indicated for those with persistent significant symptoms. Surgical options included resection of the neuroma and primary repair of the nerve, neurolysis, and neurolysis and transfer to a new location.

Symptoms of digital nerve compression in tennis players[44,52] include numbness along the volar surface of the index finger of the racquet hand and an abnormal sweat pattern, especially in players who have recently started playing or who have recently increased their amount of playing. Physical findings usually include calluses over the second metacarpal head, which implies rubbing of the digital nerve between the fixed bone and the racquet handle. Early recognition, improved technique, better equipment, and protective measures are helpful in treating this problem. Surgery is very rarely indicated.

The piriformis syndrome is not discussed with specific reference to athletes, although sporting activities may cause such changes in the piriformis muscle that significantly contribute to the development of the syndrome. Repetitive motion and loading, muscular hypertrophy, direct trauma, decreased flexibility, and dynamic compression have all been implicated in nerve entrapment of the sports participants. Hunter and Poole[53] discuss differential diagnoses for this syndrome and report that the compression of the sciatic nerve beneath the piriformis can cause similar symptoms. Runners and dancers often experience pain in their buttocks, which is indicative of the piriformis syndrome. Inflexibility of the muscle with an internal rotation contracture of the hip as well as endurance and dancing activities[54] can produce a chronic strain. Muscular hypertrophy may cause the piriformis syndrome, as seen in two cases from the editors' practice. A top 100-m hurdle runner was treated for several months for undefined pain in the buttocks. The initial diagnosis of piriformis syndrome was later clinically confirmed. Nonoperative treatment comprising rest from activity for 15 days, nonsteroidal, anti-inflammatory medication, and an aggressive program of stretching and flexibility exercises resulted in the disappearance of the symptoms. However, a top professional football player also suffering from the piriformis syndrome did not respond to nonoperative treatment and was surgically treated by a dissection of the piriformis tendon attachment. On the second day following surgery, the patient reported pain relief. The hip had pain-free range of motion. Three months later he was able to resume his sports activities to their full extent. Interestingly, no pathologic abnormality was found during surgery except for a enlarged piriformis muscle and its thickened fascia. As in the case of costoclavicular and hyperabduction syndromes, a conclusion could be made that a subgroup of athletes suffers from a dynamic neural compression within the piriformis syndrome that does not improve if treated nonoperatively. In such a case, disection of the piriformis tendon attachment is a method of choice.

In the athletic population, the **saphenous nerve** may be compressed within the adductor canal (Hunter's or subsartorial canal), or where it exists the fascia during strong contraction of the surrounding musculature, such as may occur with knee extensions or squats.[55,56] Knee pain is the primary complaint in 90% of patients.[55]

Sural nerve entrapment may occur anywhere along the course of the nerve. In the athletic population, it is most often described in runners.[57,58] Recurrent ankle sprains may lead to fibrosis and subsequent nerve entrapment.[59] Several cases have been described in athletes who sustained fractures of the base of the fifth metatarsal following severe plantar-flexion and inversion injuries.[60]

There were only few case reports about **common peroneal nerve entrapment** in runners.[61,62] Recently, Leach et al.[63] reported eight athletes, seven runners and one soccer player with common peroneal nerve entrapment. In all reported patients, running induce pain and numbness. Examination after running revealed muscle weakness and a positive Tinel's test where the nerve winds around the fibular neck. Due to failure of varying types of nonoperative treatment, all of the patients were treated surgically by neurolysis of the peroneal nerve as it travels under the sharp fibrous edge of the peroneus longus muscle origin. Leach et al.[63] reported that seven of eight operated athletes returned to their previous level of activity without any further symptoms.

Superficial peroneal nerve entrapment occurs most commonly in runners, but may also be seen in soccer players, hockey players, tennis players, bodybuilders, and dancers.[64-68] Loss of or disturbances in sensation over the dorsum of the foot during exercise is a common sign of entrapment. Occasionally, patients only complain of pain at the junction of the middle and distal third of the leg, with or without the presence of local swelling. The pain is typically worse with any physical activity including walking, jogging, running or squatting. Relief by conservative measures is uncommon. Decompression by local fasciectomy and fasciotomy of the lateral compartment has been reported to give good results.[66]

Entrapment of the deep peroneal nerve (syndrome of the anterior tarsal tunnel) has been described in runners, soccer players, skiers, and dancers.[57,58] Patients frequently give a history of recurrent ankle sprains or previous trauma. Tight, heeled shoes or ski boots have also been implicated as inciting factors.[69,70] An osteophyte on the dorsum of the talus or an osteophyte of the intermetatarseum at the tarsometatarsal joint can also press on the nerve.[71] Soccer players who sustain frequent blows to the dorsum of the feet may also develop this syndrome. Baxter and co-workers[57,58,71] described this entrapment in joggers who wore keys under the tongue of their running shoes and in athletes who did situps with their feet hooked under a metal bar. The pain usually occurs during athletic activities and subsides with removal of the shoe and rest. Running on curves may exacerbate the pain.

Tarsal tunnel syndrome is an uncommon condition in the athletic population. It has been described in runners, ballet dancers, and basketball players.[57,58,71,72] Athletes with tarsal tunnel syndrome usually present with burning, sharp pain, or paresthesias that radiate into the sole of the foot. The symptoms are intermittent and are accentuated by prolonged running. The pain is often diminished by cessation of the running, massage of the foot and ankle region, and elevation. Treatment should be directed toward identifying and correcting the etiology of the syndrome. If nonoperative treatment fails, surgical exploration and decompression of the nerve is indicated.

One of the most commonly overlooked causes of chronic heel pain in athletes is **entrapment of the first branch of the lateral plantar nerve** (nerve to the abductor digiti quinti muscle). Although runners and joggers account for the overwhelming majority of cases, this entrapment has been reported in athletes who participate in soccer, dance, and tennis, as well as other track and field events.[71,73-75] Entrapment occurs between the heavy deep fascia of the abductor hallucis muscle and the medial caudal margin of the medial head of the quadratus plantae muscle. Athletes complain of chronic heel pain that is intensified with walking and especially by running. Tenderness over the course of the nerve, maximal in the area of entrapment, is a characteristic and pathognomonic finding. Treatment is similar to that of other forms of heel pain: with rest, nonsteroidal anti-inflammatory medication, heel cups, stretching programs, and occasionally steroid injections. If 6 to 12 months of nonoperative therapy fail to relieve the symptoms and other possible causes of heel pain have been ruled out, surgical intervention is indicated.[74]

Jogger's foot (medial plantar nerve entrapment) occurs in the region of the master knot of Henry.[76] The patient, usually a middle-aged jogger, complains of aching or shooting pain in the medial aspect of the arch during running. Most characteristically, the onset of pain is associated with the use of a new arch support. Physical examination reveals point tenderness of the plantar aspect of the medical arch in the region of the navicular tuberosity. A Tinel's sign may be found. Nonoperative treatment usually is sufficient.

Interdigital neuromas (metatarsalgia) are not uncommon in athletes, especially in runners.[57,58,71,72] Patients characteristically complain of plantar or forefoot pain associated with sprints or long-distance running. The pain, described as burning or sharp, frequently radiates to the toes. Patients may also notice numbness or tingling in the affected toes. They will often give a history of many shoe changes in an attempt to seek relief. Typically, the pain is relieved by rest, removal of the shoes, and massage of the forefoot. A variety of metatarsal pads and orthotic devices have been suggested, but they are usually uncomfortable and are rejected by athletes. A small percentage of interdigital neuromas respond to steroid injections. Most of them require surgical excision.

REFERENCES

1. Strunkel, R. J. and Garrick, J. G., Thoracic outlet compression in athletes, *Am. J. Sports Med.*, 6, 35, 1978.
2. Leffert, R. D., Thoracic outlet syndrome and the shoulder, *Clin. Sports Med.*, 2, 439, 1983.
3. Karas, S. E., Thoracic outlet syndrome, *Clin. Sports Med.*, 9, 297, 1990.
4. Priest, J. D., A physical phenomenon: Shoulder depression in athletes, *Sports Car Fit*, 3(4), 20, 1989.
5. Johnson, D. C., The upper extremity in swimming, in *Symposium on Upper Extremity Injuries in Athletes,* Pettrone, F. A., Ed., C. V. Mosby, St. Louis, 1986, 36–46.
6. Leffert, R. D., Brachial plexus injuries, *N. Engl. J. Med.*, 291, 1059, 1974.
7. Hirasawa, Y. and Sakakida, K., Sports and peripheral nerve injury, *Am. J. Sports Med.*, 11, 420, 1983.
8. Wojtys, E. M., Smith, P. A., and Hankin, F. M., A cause of ulnar neuropathy in a baseball pitcher: A case report, *Am. J. Sports Med.*, 14, 522, 1986.
9. Batement, J. E., Nerve injuries about the shoulder in sports, *J. Bone Joint Surg.*, 49A, 785, 1967.
10. Redler, M. R., Ruland, L. J., and McCue, F. C. III, Quadrilateral space syndrome in a throwing athlete, *Am. J. Sports Med.*, 14, 511, 1986.
11. Post, M. and Mayer, J., Suprascapular nerve entrapment, *Clin. Orthop.*, 223, 126, 1987.
12. Mendoza, F. X. and Main, K., Peripheral nerve injuries of the shoulder in the athletes, *Clin. Sports Med.*, 9, 331, 1990.

13. Ringel, S. P., Treihaft, M., Carry, M., et al., Suprascapular neuropathy in pitchers, *Am. J. Sports Med.,* 18, 80, 1990.
14. Ferretti, A., Cerullo, G., and Russo, G., Suprascapular neuropathy in volleyball players, *J. Bone Joint Surg.,* 69A, 260, 1987.
15. Bryan, W. J. and Wild, J. J., Isolated infraspinatus atrophy: A common cause of posterior should pain and weakness in throwing athletes, *Am. J. Sports Med.,* 17, 130, 1989.
16. Black, K. P. and Lombardo, J. A., Suprascapular nerve injuries with isolated paralysis of the infraspinatus, *Am. J. Sports Med.,* 18, 225, 1990.
17. Ganzhorn, R. W., Hocker, J. T., Horowitz, M., et al., Suprascapular nerve entrapment, *J. Bone Joint Surg.,* 63A, 492, 1981.
18. Posner, M. A., Compression neuropathies of the median and radial nerves at the elbow, *Clin. Sports Med.,* 9, 343, 1990.
19. Lotem, M., Fried, A., Levy, M., et al., Radial palsy following muscular effort: A nerve compression syndrome possibly related to a fibrous arch of the lateral band of the triceps, *J. Bone Joint Surg.,* 53B, 500, 1971.
20. McCue, F. C. III and Miller, G. A., Soft-tissue injuries of the hand, in *Symposium on Upper Extremity Injuries in Athletes,* Pettrone, F. A., Ed., C. V. Mosby, St. Louis, 1986, 79–94.
21. Werner, C. O., Lateral elbow pain and posterior interosseous nerve entrapment, *Acta Orthop. Scand. Suppl.,* 174, 1, 1979.
22. Roles, N. C. and Maudsley, R. H., Radial tunnel syndrome. Resistant tennis elbow as a nerve entrapment, *J. Bone Joint Surg.,* 54B, 499, 1972.
23. Moss, S. H. and Switzer, H. E., Radial tunnel syndrome: A spectrum of clinical presentations, *J. Hand Surg.,* 8, 414, 1983.
24. Mosher, J. F., Peripheral nerve injuries and entrapment of the forearm and wrist, in *Symposium on Upper Extremity Injuries in Athletes,* Pettrone, F. A., Ed., C. V. Mosby, St. Louis, 1986, 174–181.
25. Howard, F. M., Controversies in nerve entrapment syndromes in the forearm and wrist, *Orthop. Clin. North Am.,* 17, 375, 1986.
26. Ritts, G. D., Wood, M. B., and Linscheid, R. L., Radial tunnel syndrome: A ten-year surgical experience, *Clin. Orthop.,* 219, 201, 1987.
27. Rettig, A. C., Neurovascular injuries in the wrist and hands of athletes, *Clin. Sports Med.,* 9, 389, 1990.
28. Dorfman, L. J. and Jayeram, A. R., Handcuff neuropathy, *JAMA,* 239, 957, 1978.
29. Massey, E. W. and Pleet, A. B., Handcuffs and cheiralgia paresthetica, *Neurology,* 28, 1312, 1978.
30. Del Pizzo, W., Jobe, F. W., and Norwood, L., Ulnar nerve entrapment syndrome in baseball players, *Am. J. Sports Med.,* 5, 182, 1977.
31. Fulkerson, J. P., Transient ulnar neuropathy from Nordic skiing, *Clin. Orthop.,* 153, 230, 1980.
32. Yocum, L. A., The diagnosis and nonoperative treatment of elbow problems in the athlete, *Clin. Sports Med.,* 8, 439, 1989.
33. Blousman, R. E., Ulnar nerve problems in the athlete's elbow, *Clin. Sports Med.,* 9, 365, 1990.
34. Childress, H. M., Recurrent ulnar nerve dislocation at the elbow, *J. Bone Joint Surg.,* 38A, 978, 1956.
35. Destot, M., Paralysie cubitale par l'usage de la bicyclette, *Gaz. Hop.,* 69, 1176, 1896.
36. Smail, D. F., Handlebar palsy (letter), *N. Engl. J. Med.,* 292, 322, 1975.
37. Converse, T. A., Cyclist palsy (letter), *N. Engl. J. Med.,* 301, 1397, 1979.
38. Burke, E. R., Ulnar neuropathy in bicyclists, *Phys. Sportsmed.,* 9, 53, 1981.
39. Frontera, W. R., Cyclist palsy: Clinical and electrodiagnostic findings, *Br. J. Sports Med.,* 17, 91, 1983.
40. Jackson, D. L., Electrodiagnostic studies of median and ulnar nerves in cyclists, *Phys. Sportsmed.,* 17, 137, 1989.
41. Conn, J., Bergan, J. J., and Bell, J. L., Hypothenar hammer syndrome. Post traumatic digital ischemia, *Surgery,* 68, 1122, 1970.
42. Ho, P. K., Dellon, A. L., and Wilgis, E. F. S., True aneurysms of the hand resulting from athletic injury, *Am. J. Sports Med.,* 13, 136, 1985.
43. Collins, K., Storey, M., Peterson, K., et al., Nerve injuries in athletes, *Phys. Sportsmed.,* 16, 92, 1988.
44. Osterman, L. A., Moskow, L., and Low, D. W., Soft-tissue injuries of the hand and wrist in racquet sports, *Clin. Sports Med.,* 7, 329, 1988.
45. Ruby, L. K., Common hand injuries in the athlete, *Orthop. Clin. North Am.,* 11, 819, 1980.
46. Wood, M. B. and Dobyns, J. H., Sports-related extraarticular wrist syndromes, *Clin. Orthop.,* 202, 93, 1986.
47. Siegal, I. M., Bowling thumb neuroma (letter), *JAMA,* 192, 263, 1965.
48. Howell, A. E. and Leach, R. E., Bowler's thumb: Perineural fibrosis of the digital nerve, *J. Bone Joint Surg.,* 52A, 379, 1970.
49. Dobyns, J. H., O'Brien, E. T., Linscheid, R. L., et al., Bowler's thumb, diagnosis and treatment: Review of 17 cases, *J. Bone Joint Surg.,* 54A, 751, 1972.
50. Dunhan, W., Haines, G., and Spring, J. M., Bowler's thumb (ulnovolar neuroma of the thumb), *Clin. Orthop.,* 83, 99, 1972.
51. Minkow, F. V. and Basset, F. H. III, Bowler's thumb, *Clin. Orthop.,* 83, 115, 1972.
52. Naso, S. J., Compression of the digital nerve: A new entity in tennis players, *Orthop. Rev.,* 13, 47, 1984.

53. Hunter, S. C. and Poole, R. M., The chronically inflamed tendon, *Clin. Sports Med.,* 6, 371, 1987.
54. Pećina, M., Contribution to the etiological explanation of the piriformis syndrome, *Acta Anat. (Basel),* 105, 181, 1979.
55. Worth, R. M., Ketterkamp, D. B., Defalque, R. J., et al., Saphenous nerve entrapment. A cause of medial knee pain, *Am. J. Sports Med.,* 12, 80, 1984.
56. Dumitru, D. and Windsor, R. E., Subsartorial entrapment of the saphenous nerve of a competitive female bodybuilder, *Phys. Sportsmed.,* 17, 116, 1989.
57. Deese, J. M. Jr. and Baxter, D. E., Compressive neuropathies of the lower extremity, *J. Musculoskel. Med.,* 5, 68, 1988.
58. Schon, L. C. and Baxter, D. E., Neuropathies of the foot and ankle in athletes, *Clin. Sports Med.,* 9, 489, 1990.
59. Pringle, R. M., Protheroe, K., and Mukherjee, S. K., Entrapment neuropathy of the sural nerve, *J. Bone Joint Surg.,* 56B, 465, 1974.
60. Gould, N. and Trevino, S., Sural nerve entrapment by avulsion fracture of the base of the fifth metatarsal, *Foot Ankle,* 2, 153, 1981.
61. Stack, R. E., Bianco, A. J., and MacCarty, C. S., Compression of the common peroneal nerve by ganglion cysts, *J. Bone Joint Surg.,* 47A, 773, 1965.
62. Moller, B. N. and Kadin, S., Entrapment of the common peroneal nerve, *Am. J. Sports Med.,* 15, 90, 1987.
63. Leach, R. E., Purnell, M. B., and Saito, A., Peroneal nerve entrapment in runners, *Am. J. Sports Med.,* 17, 287, 1989.
64. Lowdon, I. M. R., Superficial peroneal nerve entrapment: A case report, *J. Bone Joint Surg.,* 67B, 58, 1985.
65. McAuliffe, T. B., Fiddian, N. J., and Browett, J. P., Entrapment neuropathy of the superficial peroneal nerve: A bilateral case, *J. Bone Joint Surg.,* 67B, 62, 1985.
66. Styf, J., Entrapment of the superficial peroneal nerve: Diagnosis and results of decompression, *J. Bone Joint Surg.,* 71B, 131, 1989.
67. Styf, J., Chronic exercise-induced pain in the anterior aspect of the lower leg: An overview of diagnosis, *Sports Med.,* 7, 331, 1989.
68. Kernohan, J., Levack, B., and Wilson, J. N., Entrapment of the superficial peroneal nerve: Three case reports, *J. Bone Joint Surg.,* 37B, 60, .
69. Lindenbaum, B. L., Ski boot compression syndrome, *Clin. Orthop.,* 140, 19, 1979.
70. Gessini, L., Jandolo, B., and Pietrangeli, A., The anterior tarsal syndrome: Report of four cases, *J. Bone Joint Surg.,* 66A, 786, 1984.
71. Murphy, P. C. and Baxter, D. E., Nerve entrapment of the foot and ankle in runners, *Clin. Sports Med.,* 4, 753, 1985.
72. Mattalino, A. J., Deese, J. M. Jr., and Campbell, E. D. Jr., Office evaluation and treatment of lower extremity injuries in runners, *Clin. Sports Med.,* 8, 461, 1989.
73. Henricson, A. S. and Westlin, N. E., Chronic calcaneal pain in athletes: Entrapment of the calcaneal nerve?, *Am. J. Sports Med.,* 12, 162, 1984.
74. Baxter, D. E., Pfeffer, G. B., and Thigpen, M., Chronic heel pain: Treatment rationale, *Orthop. Clin. North Am.,* 20, 563, 1989.
75. Bazzoli, A. S. and Polina, F. S., Heel pain in recreational runners, *Phys. Sportsmed.,* 17, 55, 1989.
76. Rask, M. R., Medial platar neuroprazia (jogger's foot): Report of three cases, *Clin. Orthop.,* 134, 193, 1978.

GLOSSARY

accuracy	conformity to truth or to a standard or model; exactness
afferent nerve	nerve that transmits impulses from the periphery to the central nervous system
aponeurosis	a flat fibrous sheet of connective tissue that serves to attach muscle to bone or other tissues
caudal	towards the tail, inferior, or posterior
crura	a pair of elongated or diverging masses
crural	pertaining to the leg or thigh; femoral
dysfunction	abnormal, inadequate, or impaired action of an organ or part
efferent nerve	nerve that transmits impulses from a nerve center to the periphery
fasiculations	involuntary muscle twitches, can occur following denervation or nerve pathology
flaccid	relaxed, flabby, having defective or absent muscular tone, reflexes; a reaction to nerve damage, usually lower motor neurons of the spinal cord
fossa	a furrow or shallow depression
galvonometer	an instrument that measures current by electromagnetic action
ganglion	cystic tumors developing on a tendon or aponeurosis
heteresthesia	variation in degree of sensory response to cutaneous stimuli
Hoffman's sign	presence of this sign is shown by flicking the nail of the second, third, or fourth fingers and observing flexion. This indicates hyperactive tendon reflexes
hyperesthesia	increased sensitivity to sensory stimuli such as pain or touch
hypesthesia	lessened sensibility to touch
hypoesthesia	dulled sensitivity to touch
innervative	to stimulate a part, as the nerve supply of an organ
neoplasm	a new and abnormal formation of tissue, as a tumor or growth serving no useful function
neuralgia	severe sharp pain along the course of a nerve; neurodynia
neuropraxia	cessation in function of a peripheral nerve without degenerative changes occuring. Recovery is the usual outcome
neuraxis	the cerebrospinal axis
neurectasia	surgical nerve stretching
neurexeresis	ripping or tearing out of a nerve to relieve neuralgia
neuritis	inflammation of a nerve or nerves, usually associated with a degenerative process
neuroanastomosis	surgical attachment of one end of a severed nerve to another end
neurolysis	loosening of adhesions surrounding a nerve, disintegration of nerve tissue
neuroma	general term for a tumor of nerve origin
neuropraxia	the condition where trauma has led to the loss of nerve conduction despite maintaining anatomical continuity
neurotmesis	nerve injury with complete loss of function of the nerve even though there is little anatomical damage
nociceptive	pertaining to painful stimuli
objective	perceptible to other individuals; can be measured, seen, heard, or felt
paralysis	temporary suspension or permanent loss of sensation or voluntary motion
paresthesia	sensation of numbness, prickling, or tingling; heightened sensitivity

predictive value   the ability of a statistical test to accurately identify individuals with and without a certain trait (i.e., true positives and true negatives)

probability   the ratio that expresses the liklihood of the occaurence of a specific event

reflex   an involuntary response to a stimulus

reproducible   an event or result which can be produced repetitively

sensitivity   the statistical ability of a test to identify idividuals with a disorder from a population (positives)

sign   any objective evidence or manifestation of an illness or a disordered function of the body indicating pathology or disease

specificity   the statistical ability of a test to identify those without the disorder from a population (negatives)

spasticity   increased tone or contractions of muscles causing stiff or awkward movements; related to upper neuron lesions

symptom   any perceptible change in the body or its functions that indicates disease; may be cardinal, subjective, or constitutional

syndrome   a group of signs and symptoms that collectively characterize or indicate a particular disease or abnormal condition

tone   normal tension or responsiveness of tissues to passive stretch or elongation (tonicity: hypo- or hyper)

transection   a cutting made across a long axis; a cross-section

transposition   a transfer of one position to another

wallerian degeneration   nerve fiber degeneration when severed from its cell body

INDEX